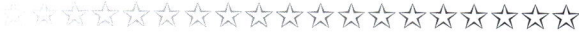

Contraception and Family Planning

Edited by

Ian Milsom, MD, PhD

Professor and Consultant Gynecologist
Department of Obstetrics & Gynecology
Sahlgrenska Academy at Göteborg University,
  and Sahlgrenska University Hospital
Göteborg, Sweden

ELSEVIER

Edinburgh   London   New York   Oxford   Philadelphia   St Louis   Sydney   Toronto   2006

European Practice in Gynaecology and Obstetrics

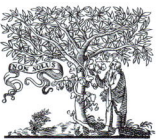

ELSEVIER

© 2006, Elsevier Limited. All rights reserved.

The right of Ian Milsom to be identified as editor of this work has been asserted by him in accordance with the Copyright, Designs and Patents Act 1988

First published 2006

ISBN 0 444 51828 2

British Library Cataloguing in Publication Data
A catalogue record for this book is available from the British Library

Library of Congress Cataloging in Publication Data
A catalog record for this book is available from the Library of Congress

Notice
Knowledge and best practice in this field are constantly changing. As new research and experience broaden our knowledge, changes in practice, treatment and drug therapy may become necessary or appropriate. Readers are advised to check the most current information provided (i) on procedures featured or (ii) by the manufacturer of each product to be administered, to verify the recommended dose or formula, the method and duration of administration, and contraindications. It is the responsibility of the practitioner, relying on their own experience and knowledge of the patient, to make diagnoses, to determine dosages and the best treatment for each individual patient, and to take all appropriate safety precautions. To the fullest extent of the law, neither the Publisher nor the Editor assumes any liability for any injury and/or damage to persons or property arising out or related to any use of the material contained in this book.

The Publisher

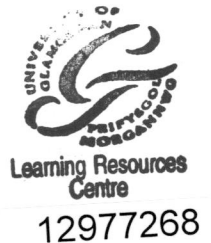

Printed in China

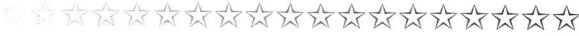

Contraception and Family Planning

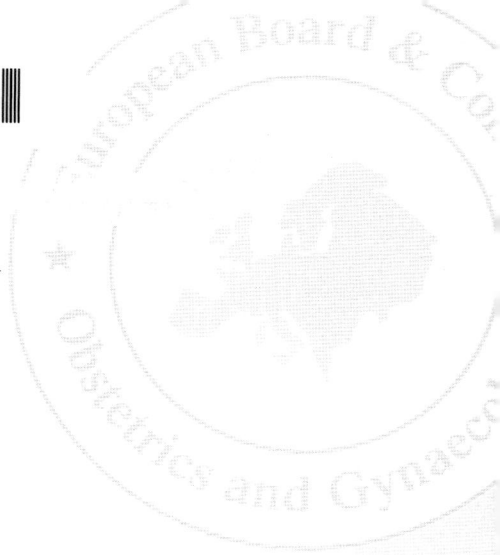

European Practice in Gynaecology and Obstetrics

In the same series

Invasive carcinoma of the cervix (Volume 1)
Volume Editor: G. Body
ISBN: 2-84299-306-3

Breech delivery (Volume 2)
Volume Editor: W. Künzel
ISBN: 2-84299-314-4

Ovulation induction (Volume 3)
Volume Editor: B. Tarlatzis
ISBN: 2-84299-316-0

Viral infection in pregnancy (Volume 4)
Volume Editors: G. Donders, B. Stray-Pedersen
ISBN: 2-84299-317-9

Endometrial cancer (Volume 5)
Volume Editor: P. Bösze
ISBN: 0-444-51361-2

Paediatric and adolescent gynaecology (Volume 6)
Volume Editor: J. J. Amy
ISBN: 0-444-51360-4

Diabetes in pregnancy (Volume 7)
Volume Editor: J. A. Van Assche
ISBN: 0-444-51513-5

http://www.elsevierhealth.com/series/ebcog/

Scientific Committee

Chairman: J. Lansac (France)

J. J. Amy (Belgium),
P. Bösze (Hungary),
M. Cabero Roura (Spain),
W. Dunlop (UK),
A. Goverde (Netherlands),
I. Milsom (Sweden),
F. Nunes (Portugal),
K. Schneider (Germany),
B. Tarlatzis (Greece),
V. Unzeitig (Czech Republic)

Commissioning Editor: Ellen Green
Project Development Manager: Lulu Stader
Project Manager: Caroline Horton
Senior Designer: Sarah Russell

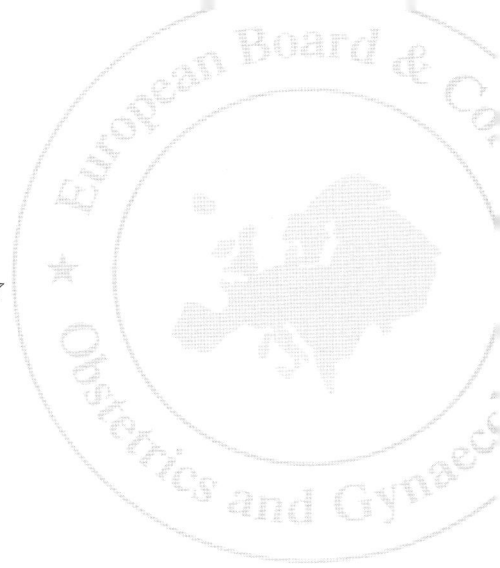

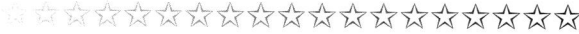

Contents

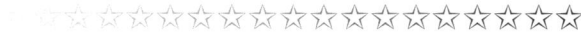

Contributors

Anne Bachelot, MD
Department of Reproductive
  Medicine
Hôpital Necker
Paris
France
Progestogen-only methods of contraception

Marc Bygdeman, PhD, MD
Department of Obstetrics and
  Gynecology
Karolinska Hospital
Stockholm
Sweden
Legal abortion

George Creatsas, MD, FACS
Dean, University of Athens Medical
  School
2nd Department of Obstetrics and
  Gynecology
Alexandra Hospital
Athens
Greece
Contraception in adolescents

Efthimios Deligeoroglou, MD
Secretary General of FIGIJ
2nd Department of Obstetrics and
  Gynecology
Alexandra Hospital
Athens
Greece
Contraception in adolescents

Kristina Gemzell Danielsson PhD, MD
Department of Obstetrics and
  Gynecology
Karolinska Hospital
Stockholm
Sweden
Legal abortion

John Guillebaud, MA, FRCSE,
FRCOG, FFFP
Professor Emeritus of Family Planning
  and Reproductive Health
Department of Obstetrics and
  Gynaecology
UCL Medical School
London
UK
Combined hormonal contraception

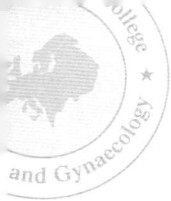

László Kovács, MD, PhD, DSc, FRCOG
Professor Emeritus, Albert Szent-
  Györgyi Medical and Pharmaceutical
  Centre
Department of Obstetrics and
  Gynaecology
University of Szeged
Szeged
Hungary
Sterilisation

Frédérique Kuttenn MD
Department of Reproductive
  Medicine
Hôpital Necker
Paris
France

*Progestogen-only methods of
contraception*

Ian Milsom, MD, PhD
Professor and Consultant
  Gynecologist
Department of Obstetrics &
  Gynecology
Sahlgrenska Academy at Göteborg
  University, and Sahlgrenska
  University Hospital
SE-41685 Göteborg
Sweden

Volume Editor, Introduction

Ellen T. M. Laan, PhD
Department of Clinical Psychology
University of Amsterdam
Amsterdam
The Netherlands

Contraception and sexuality

James T. McVicker,
MB, BCh (BAO), MRCGP, MFFP
Associate Specialist in Contraception
  and Reproductive Health Care
Abacus Centres for Contraception
  and Reproductive Health
North Liverpool Primary Care Trust
Liverpool
UK

Emergency contraception

Carl Gustaf Nilsson, MD, PhD
Department of Obstetrics and
  Gynaecology
Helsinki University Central Hospital
Finland

Medicated IUDs

Viveca Odlind, MD, PhD
Medical Products Agency
  and Department of Obstetrics and
  Gynaecology, University of Uppsala
Uppsala
Sweden

Copper-releasing intrauterine devices

Brigitte Scott, PhD
Freelance Medical Writer
Cambridge Editorial Services
Cambridge
UK

Combined hormonal contraception

Mary Short
Rock Court Medical Centre
Dublin
Ireland

*Spermicidal and barrier methods
of contraception*

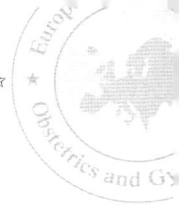

Vit Unzeitig, MD, PhD
Department of Obstetrics and
  Gynaecology
Masaryk University Hospital
Brno
Czech Republic
Contraception in the premenopausal woman

Lars P. van Dalen, MA
Department of Sexology &
  Psychosomatic Ob/Gyn
Division Obstetrics and Gynaecology
Academic Medical Centre
University of Amsterdam
Meibergdreef 9
NL-1105 AZ Amsterdam
The Netherlands
Contraception and sexuality

Rik H. W. van Lunsen MD, PhD
Department of Sexology &
  Psychosomatic Ob/Gyn
Division Obstetrics and Gynaecology
Academic Medical Centre
University of Amsterdam
Meibergdreef 9
NL-1105 AZ Amsterdam
The Netherlands
Contraception and sexuality

Anne Webb, MRCGP, MRCOG, MFFP
Consultant in Contraception and
  Reproductive Health Care
Abacus Centres for Contraception
  and Reproductive Health
North Liverpool Primary Care Trust
Liverpool
UK
Emergency contraception

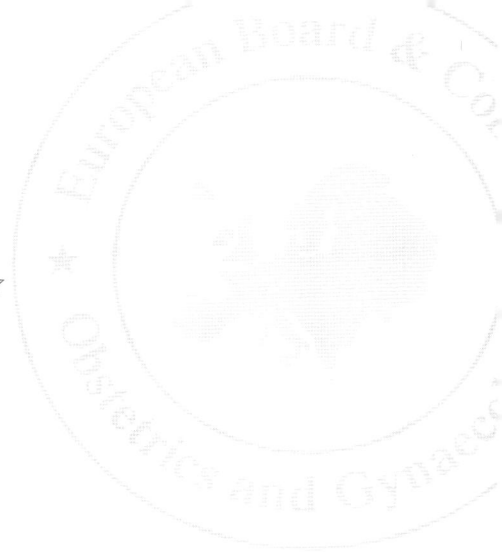

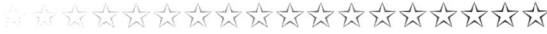

Series Preface

Why this collection on 'European practice in gynaecology and obstetrics'?

Under the auspices of the European Board and College of Obstetrics and Gynaecology (EBCOG), recommendations have been published and accepted by the European Union of Medical Specialists (UEMS) in order to standardise the training of gynaecologists and obstetricians in order to ensure quality of care and facilitate the exchange of physicians in European countries.

It was deemed that a series of books covering obstetrical and gynaecological practice was needed to provide up-to-date information for post-graduate students and the continuing education of specialists.

A common EBCOG and EAGO scientific committee is responsible for the contents of the collection. For each topic, this committee has selected the volume editor and the contributing authors, specialists throughout Europe known for their expertise in their fields. Each chapter is reviewed by external referees to assess the scientific quality of its contents and the evidence-based recommendations.

The authors describe the various types of management used in European practice, as well as the published results. They present those treatments for which a consensus exists; when there is no consensus, they discuss the key elements of the controversy.

In each book, the reader will find a review of the basic science, recent concepts in physiopathology, clinical aspects, treatment and unresolved problems or controversies, as well as the major recent references.

We would like our readers to give us their opinions on these books so that we can continue to make this collection a useful tool for students and practising specialists alike.

Professor Jacques Lansac, MD, FRCOG
Chairman of the Scientific Committee

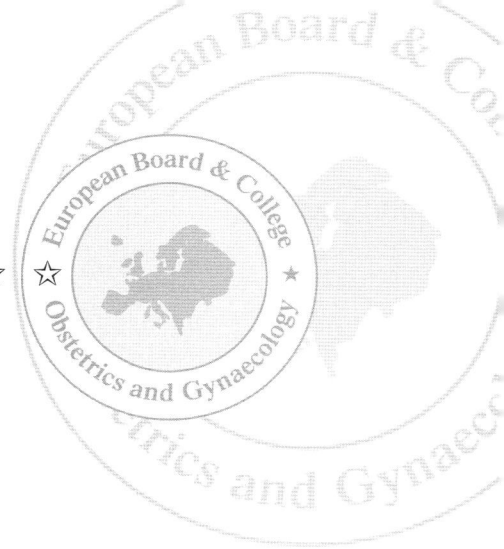

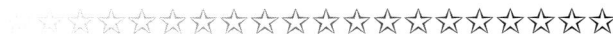

Introduction

The world's population is increasing rapidly. Population historians have reported that the population of the world did not exceed 260 million 2000 years ago. In ancient times survival was difficult and even a thousand years later the total population had not risen to more than 280 million. The world's population then began to increase and in the year 1500 it had reached 430 million and by 1750 it was 730 million and by the 20th century it had reached 1670 million. The global population had reached 2.5 billion in 1950 and 3 billion just 10 years later. By the year 2000 it was over 6 billion contradicting what many earlier writers had postulated that the Earth could not support a population exceeding 5 billion.

Induced abortion is a common procedure throughout the world. Of more than 45 million procedures performed each year at least half occur in unsafe circumstances. Unsafe abortions carry a high risk of maternal mortality and morbidity, accounting for more than 80,000 maternal deaths per year.

Teenage pregnancy is still a common occurrence in many countries and influences not only the mother and child but also the young mother's immediate family as well as society. Concerns have been expressed for the health of the mother and child and for the mother's missed educational and occupational opportunities, and possibly also for the child in the future.

With this background it is only natural to use and develop new methods of contraception, not only to avoid further consequences of the population explosion but also to promote women's health and protect them from potential early death due to unsafe abortion. The desire to control fertility has existed in many cultures for many years. In 1898 Sigmund Freud wrote the following:

> Theoretically, it would be one of the greatest triumphs of humanity . . . if the act responsible for procreation could be raised to a level of a voluntary and intentional behaviour in order to separate it from the imperative to satisfy a natural urge.

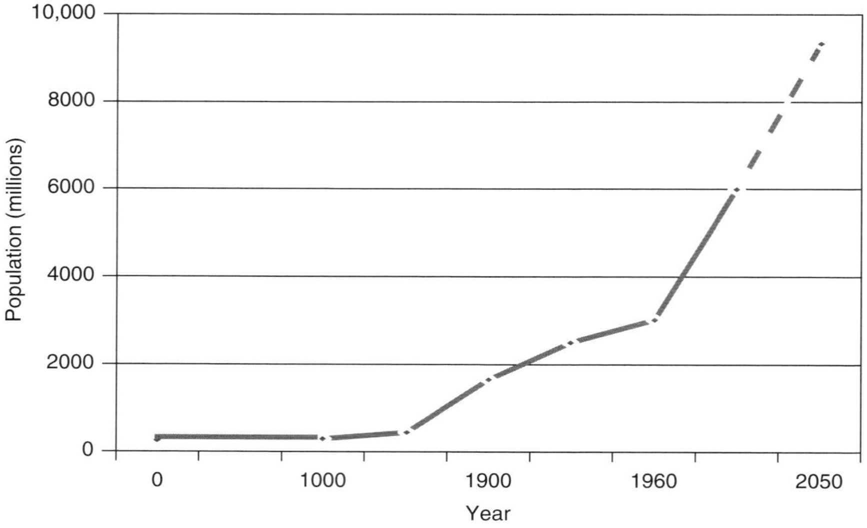

Fig 1 World population growth.

Box 1 The global perspective

● 100 million acts of coitus happen every day

● 1 million women become pregnant every day

● 150,000 abortions are performed each day—one third (55,000) of which are performed under unhygienic conditions

● 120 million couples lack contraception

● 1600 women die daily as a result of pregnancy and delivery—half of these die as a result of induced abortion

● 40% of the world's women live in a country where abortion is illegal

● 900,000 *treatable* STIs occur every day

● >30–40 million people are HIV positive and 12–18 million have developed AIDS

● 60–80 million couples are involuntarily childless

The introduction of modern effective contraceptives has been one of the most important fundamental inventions of modern times, providing the potential for reproductive health and gender equality and contributing to demographic advancement.

This book is intended as a reference book to be used by all workers within the field of family planning. The following chapters have been written by European experts within the field of family planning and they summarise current opinion on contraception methods, sterilisation and abortion. Many methods can be used to avoid an unwanted pregnancy and the text below describes currently available methods of contraception, their advantages and disadvantages as well as their applicability. However, the individual person is responsible for his or her sexuality as well as the choice of contraception. With their specific knowledge, family planning counsellors can help each individual couple to find the most suitable contraceptive method. Protection against sexually transmitted infections (STIs) should be considered when counselling on contraception. Barrier methods, especially condoms, may provide a satisfactory protection against STIs but in some situations should be combined with other safer methods. Advice must therefore be individualised and adjusted to different life situations. This demands considerable knowledge on the part of the counsellor as well as a sensitive ear to the specific requirements of each individual couple.

Professor Ian Milsom
Volume Editor

1

☆☆☆☆☆☆☆☆☆☆☆☆☆☆☆☆☆☆ | ☆

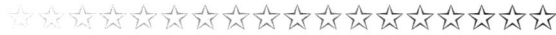

Contraception and sexuality

Rik H. W. van Lunsen   Lars P. van Dalen   Ellen T. M. Laan

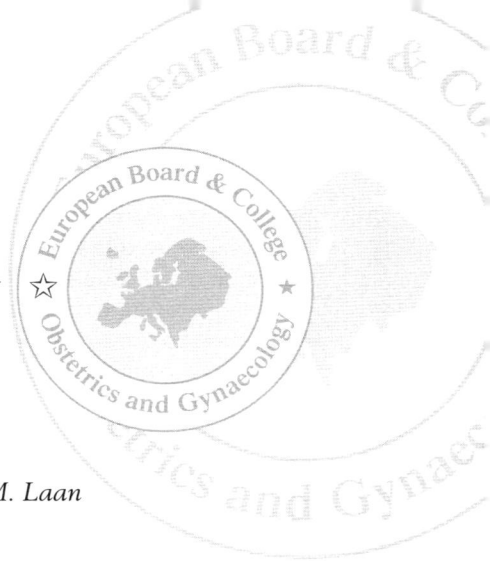

ABSTRACT

In many ways, contraception and contraceptive behaviour are related to sexuality, sexual functioning and sexual health.

The sexual connotations of contraception and contraceptive use are the explanation for existing sources of moral, ethical and religious objections against, for instance, educational activities in primary and secondary schools aimed at improving knowledge about sexuality and contraception. Both on the micro-level of the family and on a more macro-sociological level much of the resistance and hindrances to the prevention of unintended pregnancy, abortion, STDs and HIV are related to moral, ideological, cultural, religious and/or political convictions, rules, norms and values with regard to sexual behaviour.

The choice of contraceptive method is strongly influenced by hopes and expectations that the chosen method will have positive, if possible, and not negative effects on sexual well-being. In contrast to the general positive effects of contraceptive use on sexual well-being almost all contraceptive methods may afflict sexual functions, sexual functioning or the sexual relationship on a physical, psychosexual and/or interactional level. These sexual side effects receive remarkably little scientific attention despite indications that interference with sexual activity and/or functioning might be one of the main reasons for non-compliance and discontinuation of contraceptive use. Despite the recognition of the importance of androgens for female sexual functioning and of the effects of hormonal contraception on the bioavailability of testosterone, for instance, little is known about the endocrinological effects of different types of hormonal contraception on female sexual functioning.

Positive expectations with regard to sexuality and the ability to express wishes and expectations and to guard boundaries have a positive influence on the effectiveness of and compliance with contraceptive use. Relational problems negatively influence consistent use of contraceptives. Women who are dissatisfied with their sexual relationship more often report side effects as the reason for

Contraception and family planning

discontinuation of contraceptive use than women who have no sexual and/or relational problems. Women who experience pressure, threat or abuse from their partners are more at risk of unwanted pregnancy.

The existence of a sexual problem might influence both contraceptive choice and advice. In many couples suffering from a sexual dysfunction contraceptive behaviour is inadequate, either because of a negative effect of the dysfunction on the motivation to use a contraceptive method or due to an inadequate risk perception related to the nature of the dysfunction that makes intercourse impossible or rare.

To improve contraceptive satisfaction, compliance and effectiveness, at any contraceptive consultation it is not only necessary to assess the overall satisfaction and possible non-sexual side effects of the contraceptive method that is being used, but also to pay explicit attention to the experienced quality of sexual functioning and the sexual relationship as well.

KEYWORDS

Contraception, sexuality, sexual health, sexual dysfunction, sex education, teenage sexuality, double Dutch, side effects, testosterone, androgens, SHBG, relational problems, compliance, STDs, HIV, pill tiredness

INTRODUCTION

It is both remarkable and illuminating that in most medical articles and text-books, as well as in many consultation rooms, the sexual aspects of contraception are not touched upon.

In many ways, contraception and contraceptive behaviour are related to sexuality, sexual functioning and sexual health. The decision of each woman, man or couple to start using a contraceptive method is motivated and influenced by wishes, expectations, fears and anxieties related to expected future sexual activity. Moreover, the choice of one method or another is strongly influenced by hopes and expectations that this method will have positive, if possible, and not negative effects on sexual well-being. Contraceptive use is meant to make it possible to have sex without fear of pregnancy and ideally should protect against sexually transmitted diseases as well. In contrast to the general positive effects of contraceptive use on sexual well-being, however, almost all contraceptive methods may afflict sexual functions, sexual functioning or the sexual relationship on a physical, psychosexual or interactional level. The motivation to seek contraceptive advice can also be less positive. For some women in sexually abusive relationships, or other situations where they experience forced sexual contacts, the only motivation is to protect themselves against one of the possible horrifying outcomes of sexual abuse. Couples already facing sexual problems or dysfunctions when starting to use contraception may experience either improvement or further deterioration of the condition depending on the quality of the counselling and/or of the advice given. When treatment of a sexual dysfunction is successful an unwanted pregnancy might be the result if the doctor or therapist refrains from giving contraceptive advice in time.

CONTRACEPTION AND SEXUALITY—PROCREATION VERSUS RECREATION

In most articles and textbooks on contraception, contraception is defined as the instrument to prevent unwanted pregnancy. This definition is denying that prevention of pregnancy is not the primary goal of contraceptive use. If that were the case abstinence as a contraceptive method would be more popular. The main reason why most women, men and couples use contraception is to enable heterosexual coital activity without the risk of unplanned or unwanted pregnancy. From this prosexual perspective contraception is a tool to improve sexual health and sexual well-being instead of a way to prevent disasters, a tool for 'family planning' or even an instrument for population control. The ideal safe and reliable contraceptive method has positive effects on sexual functioning by reducing fear for pregnancy and does not interfere with sexual functioning or sexual activity in any other way. Most current contraceptive methods, however, are not free from possible direct or indirect negative effects on sexuality. These sexual side effects receive remarkably little scientific attention. Controlled studies on the sexual side effects of contraceptive use and of different contraceptive methods are hardly available[49] despite the strong indications that interference with sexual activity and/or functioning might be one of the main reasons for discontinuation of contraceptive use.[4] Non-compliance and discontinuation of contraceptive use are identified as the major causes of relatively high failure rates of some contraceptive methods that theoretically are much more effective when properly used.[22] In modern Western societies sexuality and procreation have become increasingly dissociated.[52] It is estimated that more than 95% of all heterosexual coital activity is not aiming at procreation. Contraception is there to meet the wishes and expectations of large parts of the population with regard to a happy sex life without risk of unintended pregnancy and sexually transmitted diseases (STDs).

The sexual connotations of contraception and contraceptive use are the explanation for existing sources of moral, ethical and religious objections against, for instance, educational activities in primary and secondary schools aimed at improving knowledge about sexuality and contraception. Although there is no evidence that sex education in schools increases the chances of teenagers becoming sexually active at an early age—on the contrary—in some societies these sex education programmes are considered as dangerous. The primary objective of modern sex education is to provide 'adults in the making' with the tools, skills and attitudes that they will need to be able to take their own mature and autonomous decisions on when, how and with whom they want to start their sexual careers; guarding their own boundaries and respecting those of others. Both on the micro-level of, for instance, the family and on a more macro-sociological level much of the resistance and hindrances to the prevention of unintended pregnancy, abortion, STDs and HIV are related to moral, ideological, cultural, religious and/or political convictions, rules, norms and values with regard to sexual behaviour. The situation, therefore, differs from country to country. Premarital sex is much debated in the United States of America (USA) while in most Northern European countries it is no longer an issue.

CONTRACEPTION AND TEENAGE SEXUALITY

In all industrialised Western European and North American countries there has been a gradual decrease in the age of first intercourse since about 1960.[42,46] Adolescents in the new millennium start their sexual careers at a younger age than those of the 1970s and 1980s. The median age of first sexual intercourse in all these countries is around the age of 17. The differences between countries in this respect are relatively small. For instance, on average, American and Swedish teenagers make their sexual debut some months earlier than their peers in the Netherlands and Belgium.[7,9,12] Both an earlier sexual debut and the general tendency of women in many societies to postpone childbearing to a more advanced age has led to a prolonged period during which there is sexual activity without any procreational intention. Throughout this extended period the average sexual behavioural pattern is characterised by 'serial monogamy'. Most young men and women have several sexual partners before they start to build a family. In this period of experiments with love, relationships and sexuality incidental sexual contacts take place in the period between two relationships when there is an implicit search for a new partner. The threat of HIV transmission that dominated the picture from the 1980s onwards did not significantly alter these behavioural trends.[7,46] To what extent teenagers, adolescents and young adults will be able to protect themselves against unwanted pregnancy, STD and HIV, therefore, is determined by the possibility of their using preventive methods when they have sex and not by illusive options, such as not having sex. This is illustrated by the observation that despite a lack of difference in sexual behaviour and age of first sexual intercourse between teenagers in different countries there are large differences in rates of unwanted pregnancy, abortion, STD and HIV. In Great Britain and the United States, for instance, teenage pregnancy and abortion rates are much higher than in the Netherlands.[2,26] Variables that have been identified as diminishing the risk of unwanted pregnancy and abortion are:[2,9,29,47,50]

- The quality of sex education in the formal (school) and informal (family, social, environmental) educational curriculum.
- The degree of openness in society and in the media with regard to sexuality.
- The communication skills of male and female teenagers that enable them to negotiate and communicate about wishes, boundaries and choices with regard to sexual, procreational and preventive behaviour.
- The accessibility of contraceptive methods and services.

The differences between, for instance, the United States and some European countries with regard to these aspects most likely explain differences in preventive success rates. In the Netherlands the climate with regard to sexuality and contraception is relatively open. The general attitude of Dutch parents and educators is that they do not like their teenage daughters and sons to engage in sexual activity at a very young age, but at the same time they are aware of the fact that their opinions will not be decisive. They therefore view it as an important aspect of the upbringing of their children to provide them with all the knowledge, skills and attitudes that will enable them to make their own autonomous decisions on how and when to become sexually active.[29,47,50] While in Northern European countries opposition to sex education in primary and secondary schools is rare and comes from small minorities in society, similar forces in the USA are much more influential. Sex education programmes, including explicit information about contraception, prevention of STDs and behavioural options, are prohibited for reasons of principle in about 50% of all US secondary schools while this is the case in only 7% of all Dutch schools.[14] In the Netherlands sex education aims at empowerment of teenagers to make their own autonomous choices based on their own emotional and sexual development. There is an abundance of convincing scientific proof that this kind of sex education does not lead to an earlier sexual debut and positively influences teenage pregnancy, abortion and STD rates.[32,36,38] Many American contraception programmes, moreover, aim at prevention of premarital sexual activity and at postponing first sexual intercourse. Several studies have found that these kinds of programmes not only fail to have significant effects on the age of sexual debut but also negatively influence teenage pregnancy and abortion rates and induce unproductive feelings of shame and guilt related to these conditions.[25,31,41] Even before their first experiences of sexual intercourse, teenagers in Northern European countries (e.g. Belgium, Denmark, Finland, the Netherlands, Norway and Sweden) more often take decisions about contraception and STD prevention than their peers in the UK and the USA. Nevertheless, even in countries with a more favourable picture overall, there are groups, such as socially deprived teenagers and immigrants from third and fourth world countries, who do not gain the knowledge, skills and attitudes necessary for motivated, effective preventive behaviour and compliance and who, therefore, are more at risk.[17,33,39]

SEXOLOGICAL DETERMINANTS OF CONTRACEPTIVE BEHAVIOUR

Choices with regard to contraception and STD prevention often are seen as one-dimensional processes within the individual. In the most commonly used models, such as Ajzen and Fishbein's theory of planned behaviour and Becker's health belief model, subjective norms and values of the individual are used to predict whether or not a preventive method will be used.[1,6] These models, however, only give an indication of the intention of the individual to use a preventive method while leaving out situational factors and partner-related variables that are located in between intended and actual sexual behaviour.

Decisions about contraceptive use and the choice of a method are very much influenced by the expectations of the woman and/or her partner concerning possible effects on the quality of sexual encounters, sexual behaviour and/or sexual functioning. Oral contraceptive use, for instance, is associated with positive

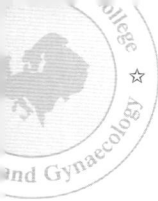

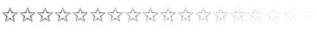

expectations with regard to sexual well-being as well as with experienced positive effects on sexual functioning in general.[44] Methods that have more influence
on sexual behaviour, such as coitus-dependent methods and natural family planning, have more negative effects on sexuality than coitus-independent methods.[44]

Positive expectations with regard to sexuality and the ability to express
wishes, expectations and guarding boundaries have a positive influence on effectiveness of and compliance with contraceptive use. Compared to teenagers who
use contraception successfully, teenagers asking for termination of pregnancy are
less positive about their sexual experiences and communicate less and less effectively about having intercourse or not, about contraceptive decisions and about
protection against STD transmission.[14] As well as relational problems, lack of
communication between partners negatively influences consistent use of contraceptives.[23,47,57] Women who experience pressure, threats or abuse from their
partners are more at risk of unwanted pregnancy.[18,20] Major reasons for not using
condoms in high-risk situations with regard to contracting STDs are the negative
ideas and perceptions of men concerning condoms interfering with sexual activity. If men do not like condoms the issue is seldom raised again and a contraceptive method will be chosen that not only does not interfere with sexual activity
but does not protect against STDs either.[60]

In general, experienced side effects and/or fears about possible health effects
are the most important factors in the discontinuation of hormonal contraceptive
methods.[23] The role of sexual side effects attributed to oral contraceptive use in
these situations is suspected to be an underestimated and rarely recognised cause
of non-compliance and discontinuation.[22] Women who are dissatisfied with their
sexual relationship more often report side effects as the reason for discontinuation of contraceptive use than women who have no sexual and/or relational
problems.[31] Many clinicians observe an increasing dissatisfaction of women
above the age of thirty with the permanent use of hormonal methods. The variables playing a role in this 'pill tiredness' have received little or no scientific
attention. As early as the beginning of the 1970s, feminists pointed out that there
is another side to the possibility of being sexually active any time: the burden of
permanent contraceptive use and of permanent sexual availability. The liberty to
be sexually active at any time has increased the necessity for women to become
explicit on how, when and with whom they want or do not want to have sex and
to express their demands on what conditions have to be met and how preventive
measures should be dealt with. In all situations where women are unable to
express their wishes, expectations and boundaries, where their demands are not
respected or where the sexual script is male dominated, the contraceptive revo-
lution has only led to a permanent availability that has more negative than
positive effects on female sexual health and well-being.[49]

CONTRACEPTIVES, STDs AND SEXUALITY

The ideal contraceptive method not only prevents unwanted pregnancy but
protects against STDs and HIV as well. The only contraceptive method that

combines both objectives is the condom.[45] In the Netherlands at the beginning of the HIV explosion condom use was relatively low and oral contraceptive use significantly higher compared to other European countries. From the mid-1980s onwards health educators were faced with the dilemma that advocating condom use to prevent HIV transmission could jeopardise oral contraceptive use. By switching from oral contraceptives to condoms unwanted pregnancy and abortion rates were expected to rise because of higher failure rates with condom use. Faced with this dilemma the double message in prevention was introduced as a tool to promote condom use as the only way to prevent HIV and STDs. At the same time an attempt was made to make the public aware of the fact that pregnancy rates due to failures with condom use are rather high and that for dual protection it was advisable to use a combination of the condom with an effective contraceptive method, e.g. oral contraceptive (OC) or intrauterine device (IUD).

This dual message, for which the expression 'double Dutch' was given a new connotation,[34] has had a certain positive effect. Condom use increased and 20–25% of all Dutch teenagers use dual protection at first intercourse and in the first years of their sexual careers. Moreover, oral contraceptive use amongst teenagers did not decrease and teenage pregnancy and abortion rates did not increase. The 'double Dutch' message has some disadvantages as well: it stresses the importance of the condom for STD and HIV protection but implicitly underlines the negative image of the condom as a contraceptive method.[59] This, together with inappropriate risk assessment and increasing risk-taking behaviour, might be one of the reasons that condom and 'double Dutch' usage rates stabilised during the 1990s and then declined at the beginning of the new millennium, resulting in increasing abortion, teenage pregnancy and STD rates. To improve condom use and dual protection it therefore seems important to direct new preventive strategies at boys and men not only in order to motivate them to take their responsibilities seriously, but also to stimulate them to practise condom application before their sexual debut and to help them to overcome their initial reluctance to use condoms, a reluctance that to a certain extent is related to the insecurity, uncertainty and clumsiness of debutants, which is the main source of condom failure as well.[34]

SEXUAL SIDE EFFECTS OF CONTRACEPTIVE METHODS

Because contraceptive use has profound effects on psychological and behavioural aspects of sexuality it is difficult to assess whether or not changes in sexual functioning during contraceptive use are a direct method-dependant physical effect or are more related to the psychological, relational or contextual impact of contraceptive use.[5,49] It has been demonstrated that side effects of oral contraceptives in general are strongly influenced by the health beliefs of both users and prescribers.[10] These health beliefs differ from society to society and particularly explain the phenomenon that in some European countries a certain method can be very popular while it is hardly used in other countries at all.

Women's contraceptive choices are strongly influenced by perceptions of the possible physical, psychological or behavioural effects of a contraceptive method.[7,43] In a German population-based survey among current and past users of different contraceptive methods positive effects on overall sexual satisfaction were reported by 44% of OC users, 11% of condom users, 28% of women practising natural family planning (NFP) methods, 30% of IUD users and 57% of sterilised women. In general, users of coitus-independent methods reported positive changes in their sex life due to contraceptive use, while users of coitus-dependent methods (condoms, diaphragm) reported a decrease in frequency, spontaneity, sex-drive and overall satisfaction. Sexual dissatisfaction during use of the method was significantly higher in past users compared to current users of oral contraceptives, condoms and NFP methods, indicating that the experience of negative sexual side effects might have played a role in discontinuation of the method.[44]

The observation that the least sexual side effects were reported by women who used male or female sterilisation not only illustrates that the lack of physical effects of the method is important, but also that the absence of a fear of pregnancy might play an important role as well, sterilisation being perceived as the most reliable method of all. Barrier methods interfere with sexual activity (male and female condom) or involve planned preparations for sexual activity (diaphragm). These influences on sexual behaviour and pre-existing negative perceptions of these aspects of usage are the main reason for not choosing these methods.[8]

NFP methods—rhythm method, symptothermal method, monitoring devices (Persona®), etc.—are not only unreliable with unexpectedly high pregnancy rates, even in a pro-NFP country like Germany,[44] but also have profound effects on coital behaviour that is restricted to 'safe' periods of the menstrual cycle. These influences on the timing of sexual activity have led to the virtual disappearance of NFP and interrupted intercourse in those countries where more reliable coitus-independent contraceptive methods are easily accessible for all and where individual or religious objections against ('premarital') teenage sexual activity and against contraception in general are less prevalent. In countries like Sweden NFP use is confined to older generations. In the Netherlands NFP is hardly used at all and a method like Persona® is not used for contraception but for spacing and cycle awareness by women who plan to become pregnant in the future.[24]

Direct effects of the IUD on sexuality have never been studied systematically. Clinical observations mention experience of painful uterine contractions during increasing arousal and orgasm in a small percentage of women. The same is the case with reports of painful lesions of the glans penis due to threads of the IUD that are cut too short. Thirty percent of IUD users report negative sexual effects of the method and there is a significant difference in sexual dissatisfaction between current and past users of the IUD, probably reflecting that bleeding problems, which are the main reason for IUD removal, are also perceived as being detrimental to sexual functioning.

Hormonal methods, due to their influence on the hypothalamo–pituitary–gonadal axis, have marked effects on circulating levels of sex steroids—estrogens, progestogens and androgens. Moreover, due to exogenous estrogens in combined oral contraceptives sex hormone binding globulin (SHBG) levels are increased[11] in the same way as has been demonstrated in postmenopausal use of estrogens[40] leading to a reduction of bioavailable (free and albumin-bound) testosterone. These anti-androgenic effects may or may not be counteracted by the more or less androgenic potency of the progestogen used. Most progestogens used in oral contraceptives are 19-nortestosterone derivatives and have more (e.g. levonorgestrel, norgestimate) or less (e.g. desogestrel, gestodene) binding capacity to androgen receptors. Some progestogens used in oral contraceptives have anti-androgenic properties (cyproterone acetate, drospirenone). Many studies have demonstrated that androgens enhance sexual motivation (responsiveness, arousability), the frequency of sexual thoughts and fantasies and some (cognitive) aspects of sexual arousal in women.[53,54]

Despite the importance of androgens for female sexual functioning and of the effects of hormonal contraception on the bioavailability of testosterone, and dehydro-3-epiandrosterone (DHEA), little is known about the endocrinological effects of different types of hormonal contraception on female sexual functioning.[4] One of the few randomised controlled trials investigating the effects of oral contraceptives on sexuality found adverse effects on sexual interest and frequency of sexual activity by combined OCs but no adverse effects by levonorgestrel-containing progestogen-only preparations.[21,37] In progestogen-only preparations with anti-androgenic progestogens, e.g. injectables with medroxyprogesterone acetate, negative effects on sexual interest have been reported.[11] It is questionable, however, to what extent these negative effects are related to endocrinological changes and to what extent they are the indirect effect of other side effects.[49] Unpredictable and irregular bleeding patterns related to progestogen-only methods, for instance, are supposed to have a negative effect on sexual functioning.[55]

In a population-based study among current, past and ever-users of combined oral contraceptives more women (12.1%) reported negative than positive (6.1%) effects on sexual motivation. For past users this difference (4.4% vs. 13.5%) was significant and significantly higher than for current users.[44]

These findings might support the hypothesis of others[4] that negative effects of OCs on sexual motivation could be a hidden cause for discontinuation or non-compliance. Further support for the effect of changed bioavailability of androgens during OC use is found in the disappearance of the androgen-dependant midcycle increase and pre-menstrual decrease of sexual interest.[13,21] Circadian rhythms in androgen levels play a role in sexual responsivity as well.[58] Hormonal contraceptives, therefore, might not only level off cyclic ups and downs in responsivity but may lead to a disappearance in daily changes as well. The difference in (anti)androgenic effects of progestogens used in OCs may cause differential effects on sexual functioning.[35,50] Theoretically OCs containing higher dosages of estrogens—by the increasing effects on SHBG—and OCs containing anti-androgenic progestogens (e.g. cyproterone acetate, drospirenone) have more negative effects on sexuality than low-estrogen formulations with an androgenic progestogen (e.g. levonorgestrel). Even the androgenic properties of OCs, however, may have an indirect negative effect on sexuality when androgen dependant skin problems (acne) increase and affect both body- and self-images of the user. Skin problems are common in levonorgestrel-only methods—progestogen-only pill (POP) and Norplant®. In levonorgestrel containing OCs skin problems are less common because the androgenic effects of the progestogen are partially counteracted by the estrogen and dose-dependent increase in SHBG resulting in a decreased bioavailability of androgens. Randomised controlled clinical trials are needed to assess to what extent the beneficial effects on sexuality of using a reversible, reliable and coitus-independent method may be counteracted by the possible negative hormonal effects on sexual motivation and responsiveness. Although there is only inferential evidence based on clinical observations and deductive reasoning that allows the supposition that there are sexual effects of hormonal contraceptives, there is no doubt that on an individual level attention to possible sexual side effects of hormonal contraception might improve continuation rates and compliance, even when changing to a less anti-androgenic OC would merely have a placebo effect on the possible psychosexual nature of the complaint.

SEXUAL DYSFUNCTION AND CONTRACEPTION

The existence of a sexual problem might also influence contraceptive choice and advice. In many couples suffering from a sexual dysfunction contraceptive behaviour is inadequate, either because of a negative effect of the dysfunction on the motivation to use a contraceptive method or by an inadequate risk perception related to the nature of the dysfunction that makes intercourse impossible or rare. In general, when treating a sexual dysfunction contraceptive needs should be assessed as well. Moreover, worries about conception or contraception should be eliminated as much as possible in order not to interfere with the process of overcoming sexual difficulties. Omitting contraceptive advice during treatment of a sexual dysfunction may lead to disruption of the therapeutic process when ambivalence about the wish for a child plays a role in the sexual problem of a couple. Omitting contraceptive counselling during treatment of a sexual dysfunction that is causing coital impossibility, e.g. erectile dysfunction (ED), vaginismus, may lead to an iatrogenic unplanned pregnancy.

Sexual desire disorders can be caused by physical (hormonal) problems and in some cases might be related to a contraceptive method.[51] In most cases these disorders have a psychosexual and/or relational background. However, when the partner with the sexual desire disorder is the woman, an OC with anti-androgenic effects may increase the problem. Moreover, OC use in hypoactive sexual desire disorder (HSDD) often has a negative psychological impact: the woman might have the feeling that she only uses the OC to fulfil the sexual wishes of her partner and that because of the OC she is permanently available. When wishes with regard to family planning differ between partners or when the feelings of the woman with regard to the wish for a child are ambivalent this might result in negative feelings about using a contraceptive method aggravating the sexual problem.[56] In these situations of dissatisfaction about using a contraceptive method in general the likelihood of experienced side effects being perceived as troublesome is increased. Discontinuation, non-compliance, forgetting pills or switching to a less-reliable method as a result of these feelings may lead to unintended pregnancy and abortion.[28] When the sexual desire disorder is related to the dissatisfaction of the woman with one-sided intercourse-orientated behaviour of the man, the choice of a non-permanent coitus-dependant method (e.g. condom) might be helpful.[58]

In female sexual arousal disorders (FSAD) and orgasmic problems possible anti-androgenic effects of hormonal contraceptives should be taken into account as well.[27] Orgasmic pain can be caused by an IUD due to painful uterine contractions. The main cause of dyspareunia is a lack of arousal and lubrication in combination with situational (vaginistic) or more permanent (hypertonic) pelvic floor hyperactivity. In cases where this results in chronic aspecific vulvar dysaesthesia (vulvar vestibulitis syndrome) the condition might worsen in hypo-estrogenic situations (pre-menstrual, progestogen-only methods, low-dose estrogen OCs, postmenopausal). In these situations, local estrogens or in the case of OC use switching to a higher dose of EE might be helpful.

The primary objective of the treatment of sexual dysfunctions that create coital impossibility, e.g. ED, vaginismus, extreme premature ejaculation (PE), is not always to be able to choose to have intercourse or not. Procreational wishes are the main reason for seeking help for many couples who present themselves many years after onset of the problem. These couples have a satisfactory sex life despite the impossibility of coitus. In any case the two possible objectives for treatment, intercourse and pregnancy, should be assessed and separated. If the couple chooses to try to solve the sexual dysfunction first, trying to conceive should be postponed and advice should be given about the use of a coitus-independent contraceptive method. If the couple not only wants to solve the sexual problem but also wants to conceive as soon as possible treatment of the sexual dysfunction can be combined with a non-sexual form of reproduction as long as anxieties about pregnancy and/or delivery are not a cause of the sexual dysfunction. In most of these cases the couple can be advised to start with at-home homologue self-insemination.[15] When primary vaginismus is the cause of infertility some women will have to start a desensitisation programme in order to be able to introduce a small syringe. Studies have shown that in these cases there is no increased obstetrical and perinatal morbidity for mother and child.[16] If solving the coital impossibility is the main motivation for seeking help and the couple has no, or at least no urgent, wish for a child contraceptive advice should be given and the couple should be counselled about the far from marginal risk of pregnancy when ejaculation occurs 'ante portas'.

CONCLUSION

The primary objective of contraception is to create the possibility of enjoying heterosexual coital activity without risk of unwanted pregnancy. Satisfaction about the contraceptive method used is one of the variables influencing the experienced quality of the sexual life of women and men. To improve contraceptive

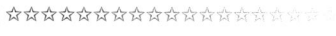

satisfaction, compliance and effectiveness it is therefore necessary that any contraceptive consultation not only assesses the overall satisfaction and possible non-sexual side effects of the contraceptive method that is being used, but also explicitly pays attention to the experienced quality of sexual functioning and the sexual relationship. If there are sexual problems or a sexual dysfunction occurs this should be assessed whether or not the contraceptive method used has a causal relationship with the dysfunction or is a sustaining factor. If necessary a change of method, preparation or dosage should be advised. During each consultation because of a contraceptive problem it should be evaluated to what extent the perception of this problem is influenced by psychosexual and/or relational factors because a woman who sees intercourse for her husband's pleasure alone is more likely to suffer from side effects than one who can see such effects as a small price to pay for her own pleasure and fulfilment.[60] Women and men choosing a preventive method will do so with possible effects on their perception of sexuality in mind. To be able to make a tailor-made choice a wide variety of methods should be available and accessible with the least possible medical interference. Over-the-counter availability of methods that do not need medical assessment does not provoke risk behaviour but enables women and men to reduce their risks.[3,19,30]

References

1. Ajzen I, Fishbein M 1980 Understanding attitudes and predicting behavior. Prentice Hall, Englewood Cliffs
2. Alan Gutmacher Institute (AGI) 1999 Sharing responsibility: women, society and abortion world wide. AGI, New York
3. Aubeny E 2004 Characteristics and use of the day after pill in France [Caractéristiques des utilisatrices de pilule du lendemain, en France]. Gynécologie Obstétrique & Fertilité 32:373–374
4. Bancroft J, Sartorius N 1990 The effects of oral contraceptives on well-being and sexuality. Oxford Review of Reproductive Biology 12:57–92
5. Bancroft J 2000 Influence of contraceptive methods on sexual function. Paper presented at the 6th Congress of the European Society of Contraception. Book of Abstracts. European Journal of Contraception and Reproductive Health Care 5(suppl 1):34
6. Becker M H, Maiman L A 1975 Sociobehavioral determinants of compliance with health and medical care recommendations. Medical Care 13:10–24
7. Bozon M, Kontula O 1998 Sexual initiation and gender in Europe: a cross-cultural analysis of trends in the 20th century. In: Hubert M, Bajos N, Sandfort T (eds)

Sexual behavior and HIV/AIDS in Europe. Taylor & Francis, London
8. Browne J, Minichiello V 1994 The condom: why more people don't put it on. Social Health Illness 16:239–251
9. Brugman E, Goedhart H, Vogels T, Zessen G van 1995 Jeugd en Sex 95. SWP, Utrecht
10. Burkham R T 1999 Compliance and other issues in contraception. International Journal of Fertility and Women's Medicine 44:234–240
11. Casson P R, Elkind-Hirsch K E, Buster J E 1997 Effect of postmenopausal estrogen replacement therapy on circulating androgens. Obstetrics and Gynecology 90:995–998
12. Creatsas G, Vekemans M, Horesji J et al 1995 Adolescent sexuality in Europe: a multicentric study. Adolescent Pediatric Gynecology 8:59–63
13. Dennerstein L, Gotts G, Brown J B, Morse C A, Farley T M M, Dinal A 1994 The relationship between the menstrual cycle and female sexual interest in women with pmc complaints and volunteers. Psychoneuroendocrinology 19:293–304
14. Doef S van der 1999 Why is sex education necessary? In: Lunsen R H W van, Unzeitig V, Creatsas G (eds) Contraceptive choices and realities. Parthenon, New York

15. Drenth J J, Andriessen S, Heringa M P 1996 Connections between primary vaginismus and procreation. Journal of Psychosomatic Obstetrics and Gynecology 17:195–201

16. Drenth J J 1988 Vaginismus and the desire for a child. Journal of Psychosomatic Obstetrics and Gynecology 9:125–137

17. Enk W J J van, Gorissen W H M, Enk A van 2000 Teenage pregnancy and ethnicity in the Netherlands: frequency and obstetric outcome. The European Journal of Contraception and Reproductive Health Care 5:77–84

18. Evins G, Chescheir N 1996 Prevalence of domestic violence among women seeking abortion services. Women's Health Issues 6:204–210

19. Fairhurst K, Ziebland S, Wyke S, Seaman P, Glasier A 2004 Emergency contraception: why can't you give it away? Qualitative findings from an evaluation of advance provision of emergency contraception. Contraception 70:25–29

20. Glander S S, Moore M L, Michielutte R et al 1998 The prevalence of domestic violence among women seeking abortion. Obstetrics & Gynecology 9:1002–1006

21. Graham C A, Ramos R, Bancroft J, Maglaya C, Farley T M M 1995 The effects of steroidal contraceptives on the well-being and sexuality of women: a double-blind, placebo-controlled, two-centre study of combined and progestogen only methods. Contraception 52:363–369

22. Hillard A P J 1992 Oral contraceptive non compliance: the extent of the problem. Advances in Contraception 8(suppl 1): 13–20

23. Ingelhammer I, Möller B, Svanberg B et al 1994 The use of contraceptive methods among women seeking a legal abortion. Contraception 50:142–152

24. Janssen C J M, Lunsen R H W van 2000 Profile and opinions of the female Persona user in the Netherlands. European Journal of Contraception and Reproductive Health Care 5: 141–146

25. Jemmott J B, Jemmott L S, Fong G T 1998 Abstinence and safer sex: HIV risk-education interventions for African American adolescents. Journal of the American Medical Association 297:1529–1536

26. Jones E, Forrest J D, Goldman N et al 1986 Teenage pregnancy in industrialised countries. Yale University Press, New Haven

27. Kaplan H S, Owett T 1993 The female androgen-deficiency syndrome. Journal of Sexual and Marital Therapy 19:3–24

28. Kero A, Lalos A 2000 Ambivalence—a logical response to legal abortion: a prospective study among women and men. Journal of Psychosomatic Obstetrics and Gynecology 21:81–91

29. Ketting E, Visser A 1994 Contraception in the Netherlands: the low abortion rate explained. Patient Education and Counseling 3:161–171

30. Killick S R, Irving G 2004 A national study examining the effect of making emergency hormonal contraception available without prescription. Human Reproduction 19:553–557

31. Kirby D, Korpi M, Barth R P et al 1997 The impact of the postponing sexual involvement curriculum among youth in California. Family Planning Perspectives 29:100–108

32. Kirby P, Short J, Collins V et al 1994 School-based programmes to reduce sexual risk behaviours: a review of effectiveness. Public Health Reports 109:339–360

33. Lamur H, Malekan B, Morsink M et al 1990 Caraïbische vrouwen en anticonceptie. Eburon, Delft

34. Lunsen R H W van, Laan E 1997 Sex, hormones and the brain. The European Journal of Contraception and Reproductive Health Care 2:247–251

35. Lunsen R H W van 1992 Double Dutch: the double message in prevention. In: Creatsas G, Serfaty D (eds) Proceedings of the 2nd Congress of the European Society for Contraception. ESC, Athens

36. Marsiglio W, Mott F L 1986 Impact of sex education on sexual activity, contraceptive use and premarital pregnancy among American teenagers. Family Planning Perspectives 18:151–152

37. McCoy N L, Matyas J R 1996 Oral contraceptives and sexuality in university women. Archives of Sexual Behavior 25:73–90

38. Mitchell-Di Censo A, Thoma B H, Devlin M E et al 1997 Evaluation of an educational programme to prevent adolescent pregnancy. Health Education Behavior 24:300–312

39. Mouthaan I, Neef M de 1992 Een Marokkaanse vrouw regelt dat zelf. Eburon, Delft

40. Murphy A A, Cropp C S, Smith B S et al 1900 Effect of low-dose oral contraceptives on gonadotropins, androgens and sex

hormone binding globulin in non-hirsute women. Fertility and Sterility 53:35–39

41. Oakly A, Fullerton D, Holland J et al 1995 Sexual health education interventions for young people: a methodological review. British Medical Journal 310:158–162

42. Oddens B 1996 Determinants of contraceptive use (thesis); national population-based studies in various West European countries. Eburon, Delft

43. Oddens B J 1997 Determinants of contraceptive use among women of reproductive age in Great Britain and Germany II, psychological factors. Journal of Biosocial Science 29:437–470

44. Oddens B J 1999 Women's satisfaction with birth control: a population survey of physical and psychological effects of oral contraceptives, intrauterine devices, condoms, natural family planning and sterilization among 1466 women. Contraception 59:277–286

45. Population Information Programme 1990 Condoms now more than ever. Population reports, H-811. The Johns Hopkins University, Baltimore

46. Rademaker J 1990 De eerste kennismaking met anticonceptie. Eburon, Delft

47. Rademaker J 1999 Determinants of effective contraceptive behavior. In: Lunsen R H W van, Unzeitig V, Creatsas G (eds) Contraceptive choices and realities. Parthenon, New York

48. Ramakers M J, Lunsen R H W van 1997 Vulvodynie veroorzaakt door vulvair vestibulitis syndroom. Nederlands Tijdschrift voor Geneeskunde 141:2100–2105 (English summary)

49. Robinson S A, Dowell M, Pedulla D, McCauley L 2004 Do the emotional side-effects of hormonal contraceptives come from pharmacologic or psychological mechanisms? Medical Hypotheses 63:268–273

50. Ruusuvaara L, Johansson E D B 1999 Contraceptive strategies for young women in the 21st century. The European Journal of Contraception and Reproductive Health Care 4: 255–263

51. Segraves R T 1988 Hormones and libido. In: Leiblum S R, Rosen R (eds) Sexual desire disorders. Guilford, New York

52. Senanayke P 1999 Family planning perspectives at the beginning of the next century. European Journal of Contraception and Reproductive Health Care 4:202–211

53. Sherwin B 1988 Estrogen and/or androgen replacement therapy and cognitive functioning in surgically menopausal women. Psychoneuro-endocrinology 13:345–357

54. Sherwin B B, Gelfand M M 1987 The role of androgen in the maintenance of sexual functioning in oophorectomized women. Psychosomatic Medicine 49:397–409

55. Speroff L, Glass R H, Kase N G 1999 Clinical gynecologic endocrinology and infertility, 6th edn. Lippincott Williams & Williams, Philadelphia

56. Stam N E 1999 Why baby why? The decision making process in ambivalent childwish. In: Lunsen R H W van, Unzeitig V, Creatsas G (eds) Contraceptive choices and realities. Parthenon, New York

57. Sundby J, Svanemyr J, Maehre T 1999 Avoiding unwanted pregnancy—the role of communication, information and knowledge in the use of contraception among young Norwegian women. Patient Education and Counseling 38:11–19

58. Tuiten A, Honk J van, Koppeschaar H et al 2000 Time course of effects on testosterone administration on sexual arousal in women. Archives of General Psychiatry 57:149–153

59. Tunnadine P 1992 Insight into troubled sexuality. Contraception, unconscious factors. Chapman and Hall, London

60. Wight D 1992 Impediments to safer heterosexual sex: a review of research with young people. AIDS Care 4:11–12

2

☆ ☆ ☆ ☆ ☆ ☆ ☆ ☆ ☆ ☆ ☆ ☆ ☆ ☆ ☆ ☆ ☆ ☆ ☆

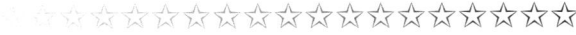

Combined hormonal contraception

John Guillebaud   Brigitte Scott

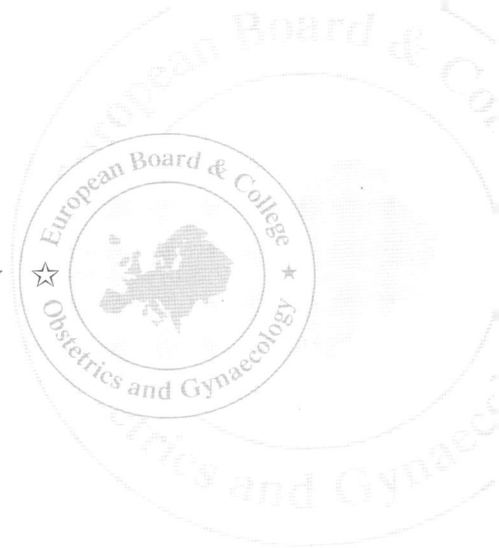

ABSTRACT

Provided the combined oral contraceptive (COC) is taken correctly, absorbed normally and its metabolism not increased by another medication, it is highly reliable, acceptable and suitable for most women. With its menstrual benefits, ready reversibility and independence from intercourse, it is particularly indicated for—and will have the lowest circulatory risks and fewest adverse side effects in—healthy motivated young women who do not smoke. It will also provide significant *benefits* to their general health. Although the risks associated are undeniable and should not be ignored, their incidence is low. Safety and likely compliance can both be increased by:

- offering the COC primarily to healthy women;
- carefully supervising those who do have risk factors or diseases;
- making time to explain, preserving autonomy of the informed 'user-chooser';
- issuing products with the least known impact on relevant metabolism;
- during follow-up: monitoring changes in risk circumstances (e.g. elective surgery) or new diagnoses, drug interactions, blood pressure and above all headache pattern; and being available for the user's questions or concerns.

KEYWORDS

Combined oral contraception, combined pill, estrogen, ethinylestradiol, phasic preparations, progestogen(s), the pill, tricycle regimen, contraceptive patch, vaginal ring.

INTRODUCTION

The use of ovarian and placental extracts from pregnant animals in fertility control was first advocated by Haberlandt in 1921. Sixteen years later, Kurzrok reported that ovarian estrone inhibited ovulation during treatment for dysmenorrhoea, and highlighted the potential role of this hormone in contraception. Development of the oral contraceptive pill accelerated in the 1950s when the potent orally active progestogens norethynodrel and norethisterone became available. Pincus conducted a screening programme of contraceptive steroids in animals, which led to development of the first oral contraceptive pill. Trials of this pill in humans were first conducted in Puerto Rico in January 1957.

The first contraceptive pills were thought to contain only progestogen and produced good cycle control. However, when they were purified the cycle control deteriorated. The impurity was identified as the estrogen, mestranol. The first combined oral contraceptive (COC), Enovid, therefore contained both norethynodrel and mestranol. This pill was approved for use in the USA in 1959 and in the UK in 1961. Although Enovid was initially considered to be associated with only minor side effects, estrogen-dose-related cardiovascular problems (primarily venous or arterial thrombosis) were reported with the pill in 1969.

Later there were various positive and negative reports regarding COCs and cancer. In 1995, some newer progestogens were reported to increase the risk of venous thromboembolism relative to levonorgestrel and norethisterone, which caused a major 'pill-scare' in Europe. Unfortunately, the medical community and the public have been far slower to recognise the non-contraceptive benefits of COCs, which have always received far less public attention.

Over 200 million women worldwide have taken the pill since it first became available, and about 70 million are current users. In a UK survey, 95% of randomly-selected women under 30 had given the pill a try, at least for a few months, and in developed countries up to 40% of all women of reproductive age take the pill. The exception is Japan where the COC was only licensed (along with Viagra® . . .) in 1999.

PREPARATIONS

STEROID HORMONE CONTENT AND BRIEF PHARMACOLOGY[12]

The composition of the estrogen–progestogen combined pill has changed greatly since its introduction. The dose by mass of both steroid hormones has been reduced; estrogen in some formulations by a factor of 10 and progestogen by up to a factor of 20. In addition, ethinylestradiol (EE) has generally superseded the less potent mestranol. In association with other short- and long-term risk factors, ethinylestradiol has the potential, dose-dependently, to increase the risk of venous thromboembolism (VTE). Therefore the dose of this estrogen in a COC is usually limited to 15–35 μg. Although estradiol and other natural estrogens are probably associated with somewhat lower thrombotic risk, when taken orally in the reproductive years they do not provide adequate cycle control or reliable inhibition of ovulation.

The currently used progestogens are all derivatives of 19-nortestosterone and some of them have been classified as second or third generation progestogens. The 'second generation' progestogens are norethisterone (NET); norethisterone acetate; etynodiol diacetate and levonorgestrel (LNG). 'Third generation' progestogens are primarily desogestrel (DSG) and gestodene (GSD). Compared with levonorgestrel, DSG and GSD have a higher affinity for the progesterone receptor and are therefore more efficacious at inhibiting ovulation and producing good cycle control at lower doses. They also have a lower affinity for androgen receptors. As measured by their effects on sex hormone binding globulin[18] and now also on important factors relevant to coagulation (e.g. Protein S deficiency and activated Protein C resistance[12]), LNG and NET are functionally more anti-estrogenic than DSG, GSD *and also the other progestogens used in* COC *combinations with ethinylestradiol,*[12,18] see below.

Venous thromboembolism. There is therefore now some biological (metabolic) plausibility to the 'pill-scare' of 1995–6 that was triggered by reports of lower VTE risk in users of LNG- and NET-containing COCs published by WHO and others.[5,26] Other newer progestogens such as norgestimate (NGM, of which 20% is metabolised to levonorgestrel), cyproterone acetate (CPA), dienogest (DNG), and drospirenone (DSP) are not usually put in the third generation class, which has become a term of abuse. Indeed, this classification into 'generations' could usefully be abandoned. CPA, DNG and DSP are anti-androgenic, which in combination with EE gives them a useful beneficial effect on acne, but their relative estrogen-dominance makes them intrinsically unlikely to have the lower risk of VTE reported for combinations of EE plus LNG. Indeed, until proved otherwise, all the non-LNG/non-NET progestogens should be seen as being in the same VTE risk category as GSD- and DSG-containing products, see above.

Arterial disease. On the other hand, low-dose estrogen-dominant pills such as those containing DSG and GSD are generally associated with fewer effects on carbohydrate and lipid metabolism; high-density lipoprotein concentrations are increased and low density lipoprotein (LDL-C) and insulin concentrations are decreased, compared with pills containing levonorgestrel. Through the 1980s and early 1990s, these metabolic differences were expected to be associated with a reduction in the risk of arterial wall disease and hypertension. There is now some epidemiological evidence to support this, for example the risk of acute myocardial infarction (AMI)[22] was not increased in users of these formulations, but among smokers was significantly increased in users of LNG-containing pills. However, an earlier paper, Dunn et al,[10] failed to show that third generation progestogens confer these arterial risk advantages over the older preparations.

All studies agree on one point, however, that all COC pill formulations are free of any significant AMI risk unless the woman also smokes or has another recognised arterial disease risk factor[25,26] (see also below).

PILL REGIMENS

Combined oral contraceptives are available in monophasic, biphasic and triphasic formulations. The brand names used are very numerous, both in Europe and beyond, hence the website of the International Planned Parenthood Federation is invaluable in listing equivalent formulations worldwide [www.ippf.org.uk].

Monophasic preparations are the most widely used, containing 15–35 μg ethinylestradiol. Very few preparations in Europe contain 50 μg estrogen.

The triphasic regimen was designed to reduce the total dose of steroids over 21 days and to mimic the fluctuations in estrogen and progesterone that occur during the menstrual cycle. Triphasic preparations produce a more 'normal-looking' endometrium. However, long-term use of these COCs (i.e. more than six months) does not appear to produce better cycle control compared with monophasic pills.

Phasic preparations provide early cycle control and are a useful second-line alternative when breakthrough bleeding (BTB) does not settle. However, they are more complicated to use than monophasic preparations and sometimes produce more cyclical symptomatology.[12]

MODE OF ACTION

Combined oral contraceptives act both centrally and peripherally. They produce the following contraceptive effects, of which the first two are the best established,[12] indeed the importance of the third mechanism appears to be negligible:

1. Inhibition of ovulation—the estrogen component inhibits follicle stimulating hormone (FSH) secretion, which suppresses follicle growth; the progestogen component inhibits the surge in luteinising hormone (LH), thereby preventing ovulation.
2. Alteration in cervical mucus—COCs at all doses cause the mucus to become scanty, viscous and cellular, impairing sperm transport and penetration.
3. Alteration of the endometrium—COCs cause the endometrium to become atrophic with microtubular glands and a fibroblastic condensation of the stroma. This is believed to be relatively unreceptive to implantation. The vasculature is reduced and less uterotonic and vasoactive prostaglandins are produced, which explains the scanty, less painful withdrawal bleeding in pill users.

PRACTICAL PRESCRIBING AND EFFECTIVENESS

The combined pill is easy to use, efficacious and has beneficial non-contraceptive effects. However, it is not appropriate for all couples. All doctors prescribing COCs should keep themselves up to date with developments in contraception, be prepared to discuss the risks and benefits openly with their patients, and be fully equipped to advise, monitor and follow-up their patients.

The pill can provide almost 100% protection from pregnancy if it is taken correctly and consistently, and its absorption and metabolism is not affected (e.g. by other medications). In practice, the failure rate varies greatly, ranging from 0.2 up to 6 per 100 woman years.

INDICATIONS

CONTRACEPTION

Women who require contraception that provides maximum protection from pregnancy, is reversible, has menstrual benefits and is independent of intercourse are often prescribed the pill. Healthy, young, non-smoking women who are sufficiently motivated to use the pill correctly are at lowest risk of circulatory and other adverse side effects.

TO TREAT MEDICAL CONDITIONS

The combined pill is commonly used to treat the following conditions,[12] irrespective of a need for contraception:

- Dysmenorrhoea
- Menorrhagia
- Premenstrual syndrome (best by a continuous use regimen with a monophasic pill, e.g. tricycling)
- Endometriosis (usually by a continuous progestogen-dominant product)
- Severe ovulation pain or functional ovarian cysts
- Polycystic ovarian syndrome (PCOS)
- Acne/seborrhoea/hirsutism (which are usually PCOS-related).
- Hypo-estrogenic amenorrhoea in young women.

The combined pill is also used in prevention, e.g. for women who have had an ectopic pregnancy or who are at high risk of carcinoma of the ovary.

CONTRAINDICATIONS

These are based on WHO's eligibility criteria, see Box 2.1.

Disclaimer. Any compilation of contraindications (as in Absolute contraindications and Relative contraindications below, using the WHO 2–4 scale in Box 2.1) must reflect the judgement of the compiler, as much as the available science at the relevant date. Many conditions that require to be categorised have not yet been evaluated in WHO's publication on Medical Eligibility Criteria.[27] Also, in a few instances, this author's judgement, on the evidence available and in the context of UK and European practice, may somewhat differ from that of the WHO.

ABSOLUTE CONTRAINDICATIONS[12]

(Meaning WHO 4, using above criteria.)

1. Past or present circulatory disease.
   a. Any proven past arterial or venous thrombosis.
   b. Ischaemic heart disease, including angina.

Box 2.1   Medical eligibility criteria for contraceptive use according to WHO[27]

WHO 1: A condition for which there is no restriction for the use of the contraceptive method

> *'A' is for ALWAYS USABLE*
> [e.g. COC use with history of candidiasis]

WHO 2: A condition where the advantages of the method generally out-weigh the theoretical or proven risks

> *'B' is for BROADLY USABLE*
> [e.g. COC use by a smoker age 20, or by a healthy non-smoker who has migraine *without aura*]

WHO 3: A condition where the theoretical or proven risks usually outweigh the advantages. But respecting the patient/client's autonomy—if she accepts the risks and rejects or should not use relevant alternatives, given the risks of pregnancy the method can be used—with caution/additional care

> *'C' is for CAUTION/COUNSELLING, if used at all*
> [e.g. COC use by diabetic without *known* tissue damage, or by an epileptic on an enzyme-inducing drug]

WHO 4: A condition that represents an unacceptable health risk

> *'D' is for DO NOT USE, at all*
> [e.g. COC use by diabetic plus *known* tissue damage, or by any woman with migraine *with aura*]

Notes:

1. Clinical judgement is required, always in consultation with the contraceptive user, especially:
   - In all category WHO 3 conditions
   - If more than one condition applies. As a working rule, two category 2 conditions moves the situation to category 3, and, if any category 3 condition applies, the addition of either a 2 or a 3 condition normally means WHO 4 (DO NOT USE).
2. Yet excessive caution is also to be avoided: women are often unnecessarily refused the pill when they have conditions that may actually benefit from, or at least be unaffected by, this contraceptive method (e.g. hypo-estrogenic amenorrhoea, thrush or fibroids, all being WHO 1).

(Adapted from www.who.int/reproductive-health; J.Guillebaud[11])

---

c. Severe or combined risk factors for venous or arterial disease. (*Please see* the Absolute contraindication (WHO 4) columns in Tables 2.1 and 2.2).

d. Migraine preceded by aura (see Aura with migraine, p. 34) or requiring ergotamine treatment.

e. Transient ischaemic attacks even without headache.

f. Atherogenic lipid disorders (as interpreted by the laboratory, after testing, which should be triggered by a strong relevant family history for the particular case). If the lipid abnormality is controlled on treatment, the COC may sometimes with specialist advice be WHO 3, pill cautiously usable.

g. Known prothrombotic abnormality of coagulation or fibrinolysis (neither to be routinely tested for, only if strong family history), including:

- the inherited thrombophilias with abnormal levels of individual factors
- acquired thrombophilia: development of antiphospholipid antibodies such as the (unhelpfully named) lupus anticoagulant, associated with connective tissue disorders, such as systemic lupus erythematosus (SLE).

h. Other conditions predisposing to thrombosis including:
- severe primary or secondary polycythaemia or thrombocythaemia
- elective major or leg surgery (see below)
- during leg immobilization (e.g. severe fracture)
- before and after all varicose vein treatments (medical or surgical).

i. Past cerebral haemorrhage (exceptionally the COC may be permitted after successful surgery following a subarachnoid haemorrhage), or cerebral venous thrombosis.

j. Vascular malformations of the brain.

k. Significant structural heart disease,[12] such as *valvular heart disease or shunts/septal defects*, but these are only WHO 4 *if* there is an added arterial or venous thromboembolic risk (persisting, if there has been surgery—always discuss with cardiologist, could be WHO 3 especially if on warfarin). Important examples are atrial fibrillation whether sustained or paroxysmal, or not currently but there is a high risk (e.g. mitral stenosis); dilated left atrium (>4 cm); all cyanotic heart disease; any dilated cardiomyopathy but not a past history of the pregnancy-related condition now in full remission, which is only WHO 2.[12]

In other structural heart conditions, if there is little or no direct or indirect risk of thromboembolism (this being the crucial point to check with any cardiologist involved), the COC is usable (WHO 3 or 2).

Note: Minor/uncomplicated valve pathology, including mitral valve prolapse, or after successful surgery restoring normal anatomy is WHO 2.

2. Pulmonary hypertension, any cause.
3. Diseases of the liver.
   a. Active liver disease (i.e. currently abnormal liver function tests; infiltrations and severe cirrhosis); past cholestatic jaundice if causally linked with COC (but a history of this in pregnancy is WHO 2 according to WHO).
   COCs may be prescribed after viral hepatitis once liver function tests have returned to normal for at least three months.
   b. Liver adenoma or carcinoma.
   c. Acute porphyria.
4. History of a serious condition known to be affected by sex-steroids or by previous COC use.
   a. Chorea.
   b. COC-induced hypertension.
   c. Past acute pancreatitis (if linked with hypertriglyceridaemia).
   d. Pemphigoid gestationis (formerly termed herpes gestationis).

   e. Haemolytic uraemic syndrome or thrombotic thrombocytopenic purpura.

   f. Stevens–Johnson syndrome (erythema multiforme), if COC-associated.

   g. Most cases of systemic SLE—but if in remission and with no added thrombotic risk (as in 1g above) may sometimes be WHO 3.

5. Pregnancy.

6. Undiagnosed genital tract bleeding.

7. Estrogen-dependent neoplasms, especially breast cancer. Past breast biopsy showing premalignant epithelial atypia is also WHO 4.

8. If a woman's anxiety about COC safety is not relieved by counselling.

RELATIVE CONTRAINDICATIONS

(WHO 3 or WHO 2 using WHO's criteria.[12])

1. Risk factors for venous disease (Table 2.1) and arterial disease (Table 2.2—see the relative contraindications columns).

   • These are usually WHO 2, provided, normally, that only one is present, and that it is not serious enough to make it an absolute contraindication. In the case of blood pressure, WHO assigns BP in the range 140–159 systolic and 90–99 diastolic to category 3, and WHO 4 if above these values on repeated testing.

   • High altitude. A special consideration applies to trekkers and others who plan to travel to above 2500 metres and especially above 4000 metres.[12] They should be warned that this is WHO 3—because in the most severe forms of altitude illness (should this occur) there may be thrombotic events and patchy pulmonary hypertension.

2. Sex-steroid dependent cancer.

   • A history of breast cancer is almost invariably considered WHO 4 for the COC, but after five years in remission progestogen-only methods are acceptable (WHO 3).

   • After successful treatment, malignant melanoma is WHO 2 for starting or continuing with the COC.

   • Trophoblastic disease: in the UK this is still considered WHO 3, just until hCG levels are undetectable,[12] though WHO itself classifies this as WHO 1 from the outset.[27]

3. Amenorrhoea or oligomenorrhoea should be investigated but the pill may subsequently be prescribed, and is often (e.g. in hypoestrogenism or PCOS) positively beneficial (WHO 1).

4. Hyperprolactinaemia so long as there is continuing treatment is now considered only WHO 2, for patients under specialist supervision.

5. Chronic systemic diseases (WHO 2 provided there is no summation with COC effects, see below). Inflammatory bowel disease is WHO 2, but WHO 3 if it is severe/extensive, as there is an increased risk of VTE during exacerbations and (in Crohn's disease) absorption of the hormones may be impaired.

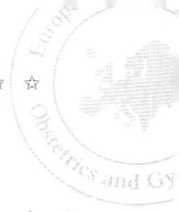

Table 2.1 Risk factors for venous thromboembolism (VTE)

Risk factor	Absolute contraindication	Relative contraindication		Remarks
	WHO 4	WHO 3	WHO 2	
Family history (FH) of thrombophilia or of venous thrombosis in sibling or parent	Identified clotting abnormality of any kind (including acquired type)	FH of thrombosis in parent or sibling <45 with recognized precipitating factor, e.g. major surgery, postpartum, and thrombophilia screen not available	FH of thrombotic event in parent or sibling <45 with or without a recognized precipitating factor and *normal* thrombophilia screen	Idiopathic VTE in a parent or sibling <45 is an indication for a thrombophilia screen if available
	FH of a defined thrombophilia or idiopathic thrombotic event in parent or sibling <45 and thrombophilia screen not (yet) available		FH in parent or sibling ≥45 or FH in second-degree relative [classified WHO 2 but tests not indicated]	The decision to undertake screening in other situations (including where there was a recognized precipitating factor) will be unusual because it is not cost effective—might be done on clinical grounds, in discussion with the woman. Even a normal thrombophilia screen cannot be entirely reassuring
Overweight (high BMI)	BMI >39	BMI 30–39	BMI 25–29	
Immobility	Bed-bound or leg fractured and immobilized	Wheelchair life	Moderately reduced mobility for other reason	

(Continued)

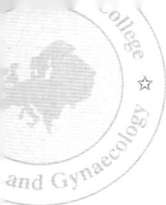

Table 2.1 Risk factors for venous thromboembolism (VTE)—Continued

Risk factor	Absolute contraindication	Relative contraindication		Remarks
	WHO 4	WHO 3	WHO 2	
Varicose veins (VVs)	Current superficial vein thrombosis in the upper thigh	History of superficial vein thrombosis (SVT) in the lower limbs, no deep vein thrombosis	—	SVT does not result in pulmonary embolism, although this past history means caution (WHO 3) in case it is a marker of future VTE risk (not confirmed). Exceptionally, thrombosis of the greater saphenous vein reaching to the sapheno-femoral vein junction, can extend into the deep system—such a history is WHO 4 for the COC
	Current sclerotherapy for VVs (or imminent VV surgery)			
	Age >35		Age 35–51	

Notes:

1. A single risk factor in the relative contraindication columns indicates use of LNG/NET pill if any COC used.
2. Beware of synergism: more than one factor in either relative contraindication column. As a working rule, two WHO 2 conditions makes WHO 3; and if WHO 3 applies, addition of either a WHO 2 or WHO 3 condition normally means WHO 4 (do not use).
3. The literature on the association of smoking with venous thromboembolic disease offers no consensus (compare arterial disease).
4. Acquired predispositions also exist through disease, see Absolute contraindications 1g, p. 23.
5. There are also important acute VTE risk factors, which need to be considered in individual cases; notably long-haul flights and dehydration through any cause.
6. This is author's classification. WHO categorises FH of VTE in parent or sibling (without further investigation), BMI >30 (no upper limit) and past SVT all as WHO 2.

BMI, body mass index; COC, combined oral contraception; FH, family history; LNG, levonorgestrel; NET, norethisterone; SVT, superficial venous thrombosis; VTE, venous thromboembolism; VV, varicose veins. (From Guillebaud 2004,[12] Table 5.10)

Table 2.2 Risk factors for arterial disease

Risk factor	Absolute contraindication WHO 4	Relative contraindication WHO 3	Relative contraindication WHO 2	Remarks
Family history (FH) of atherogenic lipid disorder or of arterial cardiovascular system (CVS) event in sibling or parent	Identified atherogenic lipid profile	FH of known lipid disorder or idiopathic arterial event in parent or sibling <45 and client's lipid profile 'borderline' atherogenic	FH of arterial event with risk factor (e.g. smoking) in parent or sibling <45 and lipid screen not available	Arterial CVS disease without other risk factors, or a known atherogenic lipid disorder in a parent or sibling <45 indicate fasting lipid screen, if available. Despite any FH, normal lipid screen *is* reassuring, means WHO 1 (contrasts with thrombophilia screens, see Table 2.1)
	FH of a known atherogenic lipid disorder or idiopathic arterial event in sibling or parent <45 and lipid screening not (yet) available		FH of idiopathic event in parent or sibling ≥45 or FH in second-degree relative [classified WHO 2 but tests not indicated]	
Cigarette smoking	≥40 cigarettes/day	15–39 cigarettes/day	<15 cigarettes/day	Cut-offs are a bit arbitrary
Diabetes mellitus (DM)	Severe or diabetic complications present (e.g. retinopathy, renal damage)	Not severe/labile and no complications, young patient with short duration of DM		DM is always at least WHO 3 (safer options available)
Hypertension	BP ≥160/100 mmHg on repeated testing	BP 140–159/90–99 mmHg	BP <140/90 mmHg	These levels are in accordance with the British Hypertension Society and WHO
		On treatment for essential hypertension	Past pregnancy-induced hypertension (if in a smoker, is WHO 3)	See Hypertension, p. 46 for pregnancy-induced hypertension as a risk factor
Overweight	BMI >39	BMI 30–39	BMI 25–29	

(Continued)

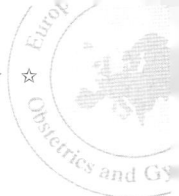

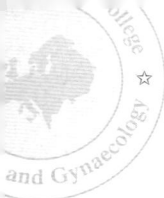

Table 2.2 Risk factors for arterial disease—Continued

Risk factor	Absolute contraindication	Relative contraindication		Remarks
	WHO 4	WHO 3	WHO 2	
Migraine	Migraine with aura	Migraine without aura plus single WHO 2 arterial risk factor (see Fig. 2.1)	Migraine without aura	Relates to stroke risk, see text
	Migraine without aura if severe prolonged attacks (>72h) or ergotamine-treated			Triptan treatment does not affect the category
Age >35	Age >51 (safer options available)	Age >40 in ex-heavy smokers to age 35	Age 35–51 in non-smokers (in smokers age >35 is WHO 4)	In ex-heavy smokers, category WHO 3 is because earlier arterial wall damage may persist

Notes:

1. Beware of synergism: more than one factor in either relative contraindication column. As a working rule, two WHO 2 conditions makes WHO 3; and if WHO 3 applies, addition of either a WHO 2 or WHO 3 condition normally means WHO 4 (do not use).
2. The pill seems to give no added adverse effect in arterial disease unless there is a risk factor. In continuing smokers, COC is generally stopped at age 35 in Europe. But WHO's eligibility criteria surprisingly permit the category WHO 3 above age 35 for smokers if <15 per day.
3. Note 'overweight' appears in both Tables 2.1 and 2.2—if it is the sole risk factor (WHO 2 or 3) it indicates use of an LNG/NET pill (i.e. Table 2.1 takes precedence).
4. Some of the numbers selected are arbitrary and perhaps too strict if they are the sole problem (e.g. the COC might actually be allowed, reluctantly, to an otherwise currently healthy 25 year old admitting to 40 cigarettes a day).
5. Numbers also relate to use for contraception: use of COCs for medical indications often entails a different risk/benefit analysis, i.e. the extra therapeutic benefits might outweigh expected extra risks. Once again this is the author's classification; some differences from WHO.
6. Check with local laboratory as to clinical significance of results from fasting lipids.

(From Guillebaud 2004,[12] Table 5.11)

6. Gall-stones are WHO 3, but WHO 2 after cholecystectomy.
7. Diseases requiring long-term treatment with drugs, which might interact with the pill (WHO 3).
8. Conditions that impair absorption of COCs, such as some operations for morbid obesity.
9. After treatment for, or during the monitoring of, cervical intraepithelial neoplasia (WHO 2).
10. Severe depression, if evidence of apparent exacerbation by COCs (WHO 2–3)—but unwanted pregnancies can be very depressing too!

INTERACTING DISEASES

COCs neutral. Conditions/disorders in which COCs are *not known* to have any effect (either beneficial or adverse) are in category WHO 2. These are numerous and are listed elsewhere.[12]

Sickle cell trait is not a contraindication to COC use (WHO 1). Both the homozygous conditions producing sickle cell disease (SS and SC genes) and COCs independently lead to an increased risk of thrombosis, which may be exacerbated during the arterial stasis of a sickling crisis, and hence according to most manufacturers the COC should never be used. Because of reassuring studies in West Africa and the West Indies and the serious risks of pregnancy in sickle cell disease, however, WHO categorises it as WHO 2 only.[12,27]

Harmful interaction. Disorders of varying degrees of seriousness in which the COC *might* have the potential to interact in a harmful way (mainly WHO 4, sometimes 3).

Though most of the important ones appear above, it is impossible to list every known disease that might have a bearing on pill prescribing. For many, data are not available or are contradictory. There are some useful criteria, which can be applied if the prescriber first makes all necessary enquiries about the condition itself, however rare it may be.[12]

Because they may summate with other risk factors, COCs are absolutely contraindicated (WHO 4) if the disorder significantly:

- Increases the risk of thrombosis (see Absolute contraindications above and Tables 2.1 and 2.2).
- Predisposes to arterial wall disease.
- Adversely affects liver function.
- Shows a tendency to sex-steroid hormone dependency (e.g. deterioration with previous administration of COCs).

But in some cases, e.g. diabetes mellitus, the added risk of pregnancy in women with the condition, or the likelihood of deterioration of the disease in pregnancy, may fully justify some increased risk due to the COC and make the disorder only a relative contraindication (i.e. WHO 3), primarily because the COC is so effective.[12] Separate therapeutic benefits (e.g. control of heavy or painful menses in someone physically disabled) may also favourably increase the benefit/risk difference.

Diabetes mellitus.[12] The combined pill does not increase the risk of this developing, although it may decrease glucose tolerance and cause a small rise in insulin levels in healthy non-diabetic women. In my view it is WHO 3 for low dose pills to be used by non-smoking diabetics under age 35, in the short term, who have good diabetic control; and if they have any other risk factors (smoking, BMI above 30), or signs of the somatic complications of the disease, the category shifts to WHO 4. Without these, as usual in WHO 3 conditions, an alternative method, such as an intrauterine device or low-dose progestogen, would still be preferable.

Drug interaction. Conditions treated with drugs that may interact with COCs (WHO 3, see below).

ADVANTAGES[5]

The combined pill is a reliable, reversible and convenient method that is independent of intercourse. Women who take the pill have more regular bleeds (or fewer or none if they so choose, see p. 43), reduced blood loss and a decreased incidence of iron deficiency anaemia. In addition, menstrual and premenstrual symptoms, such as dysmenorrhoea and premenstrual tension, are often relieved, and ovulation pain is abolished. Unlike most other commonly used drugs, COC overdose is not associated with acute toxicity, except for withdrawal bleeding in prepubertal girls, and vomiting.

Women who take COCs have a decreased incidence of benign breast disease; functional ovarian cysts; pelvic inflammatory disease (PID); ectopic pregnancy; seborrhoeic conditions (including acne) and, in some studies, endometriosis. They are also protected against carcinoma of the ovary and endometrium and possibly against colorectal cancers, rheumatoid arthritis, thyroid disease, duodenal ulcer, trichomonal vaginitis and toxic shock syndrome.[5]

DISADVANTAGES

It is not surprising that a combination of steroids that so effectively controls reproduction also affects other physiological systems. Safety issues have mainly related to the ethinylestradiol component, as this is a potent, prothrombotic estrogen with a long half-life. Levonorgestrel and norethisterone appear to reduce the risk of VTE from a given dose of estrogen (see Steroid hormone content, p. 20, and Venous disease, pp. 21, 33), but if an arterial risk factor exists levonorgestrel may possibly increase the risks of AMI (though the data are not consistent, see p. 21).

Clinical experience indicates that modern low-dose preparations still cause the so-called 'minor' side effects such as nausea and fluid retention, but are less likely to do so than earlier products.

METABOLIC EFFECTS

The metabolic effects of COCs are numerous and varied; many are similar to those found in normal pregnancy. This may seem reassuring, but it should be remembered that pregnancy has its own hazards.

Contraceptive steroids are metabolised by the liver and affect its function.[12] The resultant effects on the metabolism of carbohydrates, lipids, plasma proteins, amino acids, vitamins, enzymes and coagulation and fibrinolysis factors explain the majority of the adverse effects. See also Steroid hormone content, p. 20, above.

VENOUS DISEASE

The risk of venous thromboembolism (VTE) with COCs is related to an estrogen-induced alteration of clotting factor levels that promotes coagulation. Platelet function is also modified. There is no effect of past use; restoration of clotting factor changes to normal has been shown to occur within four weeks. The influence of the progestogen type has been well summarised by WHO.[25,26]

There are a number of established underlying risk factors for the development of VTE, including older age, obesity, previous VTE; haemostatic abnormalities, such as deficiency of antithrombin III, protein C, or activated protein C and protein S (see Steroid hormone content, p. 21); malignant disease; and acute medical illness. In addition, a spectrum of clinical settings is recognised to be associated with the risk of VTE, including major surgery (e.g. general, orthopaedic and cancer surgery, and renal transplantation), trauma, prolonged immobility or paralysis, and prolonged journeys especially long-haul aeroplane flights.

Women with congenital thrombophilia have a predisposition to thrombosis, which increases the risk of VTE with COC use. It is *not* cost-effective to screen all women for this condition,[12] but if the tests are available targeted screening is appropriate for women with a sibling or parent with thrombophilia or the history of an idiopathic thrombotic event under age 45.

ARTERIAL DISEASE

Myocardial infarction

According to the WHO's Scientific Group,[25,26] the incidence of fatal and non-fatal acute myocardial infarction (AMI) is very low in women of reproductive age. The risk of AMI in pill-takers who do not smoke, who have their blood pressure checked and do not have hypertension or diabetes is not increased by any brand of COCs compared with non-users. There is no increase in the relative risk of AMI with increasing duration of use or past use of COCs. Although the *incidence* of AMI increases exponentially with age, the *relative risk* of AMI in current users of COCs does not change with increasing age. The increased absolute risk of AMI in women who smoke or have hypertension is significantly elevated by the added use of COCs.

Ischaemic and haemorrhagic strokes

The WHO Scientific Group also concluded[25,26] that ischaemic and haemorrhagic strokes are very rare in women of reproductive age and that there is no increase in relative risk with increasing duration of use or past use of COCs. The risk of *ischaemic stroke* in women who do not smoke, who have their blood pressure checked and who do not have hypertension is increased about 1.5-fold in current users of low-dose COCs compared with non-users (and further increased with increasing estrogen dose). However, the relative risk of *haemorrhagic stroke* is not increased by COCs in women aged less than 35 years with absence of the afore-mentioned risk factors. The risk of both ischaemic and haemorrhagic stroke in current COC users is increased with hypertension, smoking, and increasing age, but available data do not show any effect of progestogen type or dose.

Migraine with focal aura. This is a specific risk factor for ischaemic stroke,[9] and hence in category WHO 4 for COC use (see Absolute contraindications, pp. 23–26, and Myocardial infarction, p. 33, above). Indeed, better prescribing and follow-up for all migraine sufferers offers real potential to reduce the observed COC-related increase in this specific risk.

Aura with migraine—some useful guidance[12]

- Aura symptoms develop gradually before the headache, last up to one hour (usually 20–30 minutes) and resolve completely. There may be a gap from resolution of aura before headache begins or headache may start as aura resolves.
- Headache may rarely be absent but the typical features of aura confirm the diagnosis (i.e. still WHO 4 for COC when no headache follows).
- 99% of auras are visual, usually involving partial visual loss, a bright scotoma. Aura may gradually spread across the visual field as a convex shape with a scintillating zig-zag edge surrounding the scotoma.
- Aura can be difficult to diagnose: *a most useful clinical sign to watch for is the zig-zag line that patients usually draw in the air beside their head with a finger of either hand[12]*–when asked to describe what occurs *before* their headaches start.
- Although not essential for the diagnosis of aura, sensory symptoms may be confirmatory. These are typically pins and needles spreading up one arm or affecting one side of the face. Nominal aphasia is less common; and loss of motor function though serious (suggesting a transient ischaemic attack) is not a feature of aura.
- *During* the headache, generalized blurred vision, 'spots in front of the eyes', or photophobia, are common and are *not* diagnostic for aura.

Avoid COC (WHO 4) if aura is present, or there are severe or multiple additional risk factors for arterial disease, or if ergot derivatives are used to treat. Otherwise COCs can be used (WHO 2 if simple migraine without aura in a non-smoker), or used with caution (WHO 3) if there is one other risk factor.[16] See Fig 2.1.

CLINICAL MANAGEMENT

Current scientific evidence indicates that the safe provision of COCs requires a careful personal and family history (with emphasis on cardiovascular risk factors) and an accurate blood pressure,[14] but routine breast and pelvic examinations are of no relevance whatever to the pill. The same applies to all tests of blood or other body fluids. Examinations and tests should be done only in the presence of specific clinical indications (see below). Women who request the pill should be informed of the issues relating to circulatory disease and cancer and should be given time to discuss any concerns.

CLINICAL HISTORY

The importance of avoiding pregnancy should be considered for each woman and the following conditions that might disclose WHO 3 or 4 conditions, or indicate use of particular formulations, should be particularly noted:

- Social factors (particularly those relating to the risk of sexually transmissible infections, STIs)
- Family history (with emphasis on cardiovascular disease and breast cancer)
- Obstetric history (e.g. pregnancy-induced hypertension, see p. 46)
- Past or current illnesses and investigations
- Current drug therapy
- All allergies

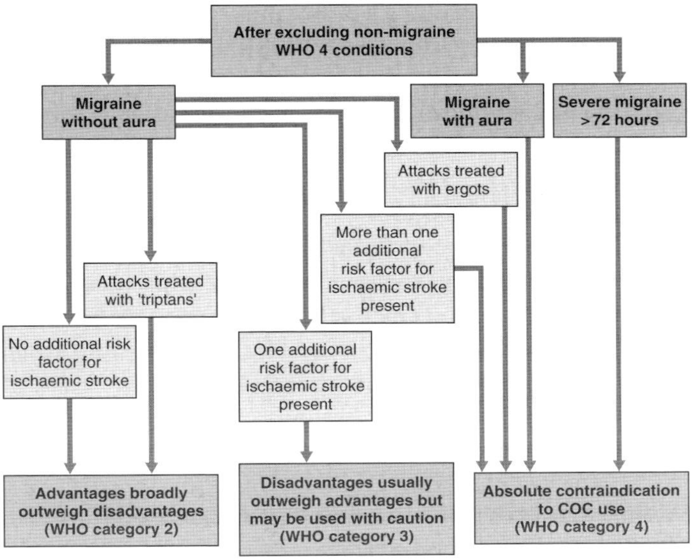

Fig 2.1 Flow diagram for COC use and migraine.
(From Guillebaud 2004,[12] Figure 5.13)

- Headache or migraine (in terms of frequency, site, timing, severity, relation to menstrual cycle, initiating factors, therapy and presence of focal symptoms in any aura, as described above)
- Acne, indicating use of a more estrogen-dominant product.

EXAMINATION

After observing the woman's general health, her baseline weight, height (and hence body mass index, BMI) and blood pressure should be recorded.

Pelvic examination is never enjoyed by any woman, and is completely unnecessary at this stage,[12] provided she has a normal menstrual history and normal last menstrual period. A recent cervical smear is not a prerequisite for any method of contraception and smears should be conducted according to the local agreed policy for a woman of that age or risk category. A baseline breast examination is also not helpful, unless the woman has any symptom or requests a check-up. She should be provided with verbal and written instruction in breast awareness.[12]

Rarely, other necessary investigations may be indicated from the woman's history, e.g. a first-degree relative under age 45 years with idiopathic VTE or heart disease usually indicates tests (if available) for coagulation or lipid abnormalities.

CHOICE OF PILL

The most suitable pill is that with the lowest dose of estrogen and progestogen to provide effective contraception, produce acceptable cycle control and cause minimal non-bleeding side effects in that individual. Doctors should be familiar with the composition of a selection of pills on the market and should keep themselves up to date with new products. Several preparations may be needed before a suitable one is found. There is no single pill to suit all women because of individual variation, especially as this affects blood levels and responses at the end-organs (such as the endometrium, see Bleeding side effects, p. 48).

PRACTICAL PRESCRIBING[12]

Although the incidence of long-term disability and mortality from VTE is low compared with that from the arterial diseases, VTE is the most common serious cardiovascular event in young women using oral contraceptives. The potential impact of this condition should be minimised by careful history taking, prescribing and forewarning (both verbal and written).

The risk factors for VTE and arterial wall disease must always be assessed *separately*. The following should be considered in conjunction with Tables 2.1 and 2.2:

- Multiple risk factors, or any one significant arterial or venous factor combined with age above 35 years, absolutely contraindicate COCs (WHO 4).
- All marketed pills may now be considered 'first line'. A levonorgestrel (LNG) or norethisterone (NET) product should be the usual first choice for young

first-time users because they will include women who are unknowingly predisposed to VTE (VTE is a more relevant consideration than arterial disease at this age) and the pills are cheaper.

- Single risk factor for VTE: one of the LNG or NET products is definitely preferable, if a COC is used at all.
- Single definite arterial risk factor, such as smoking (usually from the late 20s or after several years of VTE-free use); or uncomplicated, well-controlled diabetes; *or* if the COC is used at all by a healthy and risk-factor-free woman above age 35 years, discuss the option of using a DSG or GSD product with the lowest possible EE dose (15 or 20 µg). These pills have an unconfirmed possible advantage for the arterial walls.[22]

After (well-documented) discussion the woman's decision to have an estrogen-dominant product (i.e. any product not containing LNG or NET) must be respected. In modern prescribing they are now mainly used second-line, for the control of so-called 'minor' side effects especially acne. But the threshold to switch can be low since the difference in VTE risk is estimated as two deaths per million users per year, which can be equated to two hours per year of driving on UK roads![12]

The initial dose of estrogen should generally be 15–35 µg combined with a low dose of progestogen. A higher dose of ethinylestradiol (50–60 µg) through two tablets or a single pill if available may be required in the following circumstances:

- Long-term use of an enzyme-inducing drug (see p. 42)
- Rarely for past 'true' pill failures, which indicates unusually rapid metabolism or malabsorption.

Instructions to patients

The above prescribing protocol should be applied flexibly and always maintaining the user's autonomy. Psychology in pill prescription may be as important as physiology.

The correct use of COCs and recognition of symptoms that require urgent medical advice should be carefully explained, demonstrated and reiterated to each user, both verbally and in written form, in a patient-friendly manner. The importance of selecting a convenient time of day to take the pill and—these days perhaps by setting a reminder alarm on her mobile phone!—consistently adhering to this time must be emphasised. This minimises the risk of breakthrough bleeding (BTB) and pregnancy.

Starting the pill

See Table 2.3. The first pill is usually taken on the first day of the next menstrual period, selecting the tablet for the appropriate day of the week. Starting the pill on day 5, however, has been shown to reduce the incidence of BTB in the first cycle. One pill is taken daily for 21 or sometimes 24 days at approximately the same time. After the packet is finished, there is a pill-free interval or PFI

Table 2.3 Starting routines for combined oral contraceptives*

	Start when?	Extra precautions for seven days
1. Menstruating	Day 1 or 2 Day 3 or 4 Day 5 or later Any time in cycle ('Quick Start')	No Yes (but WHO says No) Yes[†] Yes[†]
2. Postpartum No lactation Lactation	Day 21 (low risk of thrombosis by then[‡], first ovulation reported by day 28+) Not normally recommended at all (POP/injectable preferred)	No (but Yes if COC started after day 21 as may not then prevent the first ovulation)
3. Post-induced early abortion/miscarriage	Same day or next day to avoid postoperative vomiting risk	No
4. Post-trophoblastic tumour	One month after no hCG detected	As 1 (see Sex-steroid dependent cancer, p. 26)
5. Post-higher dose COC	Instant switch[§]	No
6. Post-lower or same dose COC	After usual 7-day break	No
7. Post-POP	First day of period	No
8. Post-POP with secondary amenorrhoea, not pregnant	Any day	No
9. Post-DMPA (risk of pregnancy excluded)	Any day (if desired COC can be started well before the next injection of DMPA is due)	No
10. Other secondary amenorrhoea (risk of pregnancy excluded[¶])	Any day	Yes
11. First cycle after post-coital contraception	Day 1 or no later than day 2	No
	'Quick Start', i.e. immediately	Yes (see Starting the pill, p. 39)

Notes:

*As recommended by J. Guillebaud—WHO Practice Recommendations differ slightly.

[†]Delay into day 2 can sometimes help, to be sure a period is normal. WHO's Selected Practice Recommendations[28] are less cautious and only *after* day 5 advise extra precautions for the seven days that seemingly make any ovary quiescent. 'Quick Starts' beyond day 5 (i.e. not waiting for that elusive next period) are entirely acceptable, if the prescriber is sure that there has been no risk of conception up to the starting day (see Starting the pill, p. 39).

[‡]Puerperal thrombosis risk lasts longer after severe pregnancy-related hypertension, therefore safest to delay COC use until the return of normal BP and biochemistry.

[§]This advice is because of anecdotes of rebound ovulation occurring at the time of transfer (see p. 39).

[¶]In presence of amenorrhoea, exclusion of there being either a blastocyst or sperm in the upper genital tract can be done by obtaining a negative sensitive pregnancy test after minimum 14 days of abstinence or 'very safe' contraception by another method.

(From Guillebaud 2004,[12] Table 5.4)

(usually seven days, but this is reducible to four days in ultra-low-dose products, or with any product if indicated for extra efficacy), before a new packet is started. It is important to explain to all pill-takers very simply why the start of the next packet must never be delayed (see below).

The everyday (ED) varieties differ in that a placebo tablet is taken on each of the seven days corresponding to the PFI above, and the next packet of pills is started immediately after the last one is finished.

Contraceptive protection is immediate if the pill is started on the first day of a period. If the pill is started on the fifth day, there is a very small chance that a follicle will continue to develop in an unusually short cycle, so additional contraceptive precautions are best advised for the first seven days of the first packet. Such extra precautions are also recommended for so-called 'Sunday starts' and all 'Quick starts' (meaning that with particularly careful supervision and follow-up, the COC is commenced at any time in the cycle—often after use of hormonal emergency contraception).

Postpartum

The combined pill is contraindicated during breast-feeding. Women who choose to bottle feed their babies are usually advised to start on the 21st day after delivery, which is long enough to minimise the risk of thromboembolism but sufficiently in advance of the earliest likely ovulation (Table 2.3).

After therapeutic abortion or miscarriage

The pill should be started immediately (day 1 or 2) without extra precautions. This is similar to the advice in a normal cycle, since ovulation can occur within less than two weeks after a first trimester abortion. COCs will not interfere with recovery, nor increase morbidity.

Changing preparations

Normally the new product is started after the usual PFI. But when changing to a COC of lower dose, anecdotes of 'rebound' ovulation have dictated the (probably too cautious) advice to take the first pill of the new packet on the day immediately after the old packet is completed, or, if there is a break from pill-taking, additional precautions are advised for just seven days.

Importance of the pill-free interval (PFI)

Variable restoration of ovarian function during the PFI in many women on current low-dose COCs is well established. See Fig 2.2. This is shown by follicular activity on ultrasound and by rising concentrations of both gonadotrophins and endogenous estradiol. In a subgroup of women, a PFI which is greater than seven days will permit ovulation. Breakthrough ovulation is therefore most likely to occur at the end of any PFI that is lengthened by missed pills immediately before or after the seven-day break. According to the data reviewed by Korver et al,[15] seven tablets are sufficient to return the ovary to full quiescence when pills have been missed.

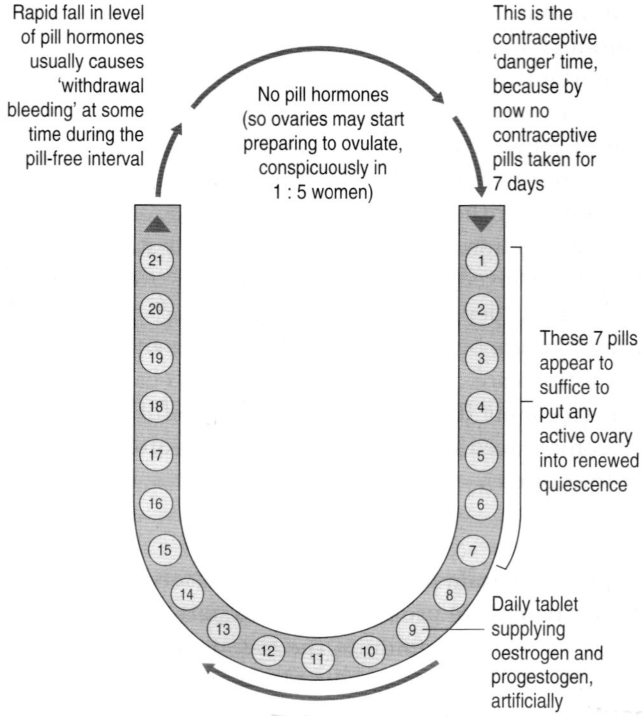

Fig 2.2 The pill cycle displayed as a horseshoe.
Note: a horseshoe is a symmetrical object and thus the pill-free interval (PFI) can be lengthened (resulting in the risk of conception) either side of the horseshoe—by forgetting pills at the beginning or at the end of the packet.
(From Guillebaud 2004,[12] Figure 5.1)

In summary therefore:

- Seven pills suffice to make any ovary anovulant
- Seven pills can be missed without ovulation (as in the regular PFI)
- More than seven pills missed, in total, risks ovulation.

WHO in its latest (2004) Selected Practice Recommendations[28] follows the principles implied by the above and Fig 2.2. Since individual variation is known to be more important than pill dose and some women can be at risk from just a one-day extension of their PFI,[13] in my view, the more cautious WHO advice for <20μg products should be applied to all COCs (Box 2.2). This means defining a missed pill as one that is a whole day (24 hours) late. Aside from recommencing pill-taking, no action is necessary unless a second pill has also been (just) missed—or more, of course.

Vomiting and diarrhoea

If vomiting occurs within two hours of taking an active pill another should be taken. If vomiting, or exceptionally severe diarrhoea, continues for more than one day, follow the same advice as in Box 2.2. If the PFI is lengthened through

> **Box 2.2** Advice for missed pills
>
> - If *more than one tablet* has been missed, the woman should also use condoms or abstain from sex until she has taken active (hormonal) pills for seven days in a row.
> - If she missed the pills in the third week, she should finish the active (hormonal) pills in her current pack and start a new pack the next day. She should not take any of the seven inactive pills if present.
> - If she missed the pills in the first week (or, crucially, was more than one day late in *restarting after the PFI*) and had unprotected sex after the end of her previous pack, she may wish to consider the use of emergency contraception: namely levonorgestrel 1.5g in a single dose, followed by return to routine pill-taking within 24 hours.

(Simplified from WHO[28] by J. Guillebaud, see p. 38)

the stomach upset, as usual this means consideration of emergency contraception—in addition to the use of condoms for the next seven days.

DRUG INTERACTIONS[12]

Certain drugs can interact with COCs and reduce their effectiveness: principally by inducing liver enzymes so as to increase metabolism and also, if the relevant bowel flora are altered by broad-spectrum antibiotics, by reducing enterohepatic recirculation of estrogen. Enzyme-inducing drugs can affect both the estrogen and progestogen components of COCs. Broad-spectrum antibiotics have a much weaker effect, if any at all, in the majority of women; they influence only the recycling of ethinylestradiol, and the effect can be disregarded after about two weeks since the bowel flora is believed to develop antibiotic resistance within that time. See Box 2.3.

Different women show great variability in the circulating concentrations of contraceptive steroids and the degree of interaction with other drugs. The individual response cannot be clinically predicted.

Broad-spectrum antibiotics

WHO's eligibility criteria actually classify these as WHO 1, meaning no restrictions on use, no action required.[27] However, at least in Europe, it is safest medicolegally to act on the basis of possibly reduced protection.

Short-term use. Women already taking the pill who start taking relevant antibiotics should take extra precautions for three weeks (i.e. two weeks being deemed sufficient for antibiotic resistance to develop plus seven additional days to restore quiescence if ovarian activity has resumed), and not have their next PFI.

> **Box 2.3** Drug interactions potentially affecting COC efficacy
>
> Clinically important enzyme-induce, drugs
>
> - Rifampicin, rifabutin
> - Griseofulvin (antifungal)
> - Barbiturates
> - Phenytoin
> - Carbamazepine
> - Oxcarbazepine
> - Primidone
> - Topiramate
> - Modafinil
> - Some antiretrovirals (e.g. ritonavir, nevirapine)—full details are obtainable from www.hiv-druginteractions.org
> - St John's Wort—potency varies; CSM advises *non-use* with hormonal methods (women need to be routinely asked re any self-medication with this)
>
> Broad-spectrum antibiotics (less important) that might interact with COCs
>
> - Ampicillin, amoxicillin and related penicillins
> - Tetracyclines
> - Broad-spectrum cephalosporins

Long-term use of antibiotics. No action. This does not indicate extra precautions in women who start to use the pill, because the large bowel flora that recycle estrogens will have had plenty of time to be reconstituted with resistant organisms.

Enzyme-inducing drugs

Short-term use. Added precautions are here advised for the full duration of the enzyme induction caused by the treatment (see below), plus seven additional days to restore quiescence of the active ovary plus elimination of the next PFI.

Long-term use. This is WHO 3–4 for the COC in the case of rifampicin/rifabutin, meaning an alternative method would definitely be better since they are such potent enzyme inducers. For women treated by other enzyme inducers, often with epilepsy or these days possibly using an antiretroviral (see Box 2.3), long-term use is WHO 3 for the COC: meaning that an intrauterine device, or the injectable DMPA is still preferable over the pill. An injectable contraceptive or the Mirena® IUS are particularly appropriate for epileptics.

However, if the woman strongly prefers the COC it may still be used. The first option is 50–60 µg estrogen (in a single tablet if available, or by advising two tablets daily) taken by the tricycling regimen described below. It should be clearly explained to her that this is still only equivalent to normal pill-taking in the absence of enzyme induction.

If BTB occurs and there is no other explanation for it (and if the woman will not accept an alternative contraceptive—definitely preferable!) the estrogen dose may be cautiously increased to a maximum of 90 µg per day.

Discontinuing enzyme-inducing drugs

The peak of enzyme induction may be several days after a drug is introduced, and liver function may take several weeks to revert to normal when the drug is withdrawn. Women who need to use an enzyme-inducer for a long time, or the extra potent rifampicin/rifabutin for any length of time, should not return to a standard low-dose pill regimen for at least four weeks. This delay should be eight weeks after any very prolonged use. As usual there should be no PFI when changing back from high- to low-dose preparations.

Effects of COCs on other drugs

COCs can lower the clearance of ciclosporin, warfarin, diazepam, prednisolone, and some other drugs. This may increase the risk of side effects, but in most cases is unlikely to be clinically significant. The exceptions are ciclosporin and warfarin, whose levels/activity should be monitored more frequently if ever taken with COCs (or after hormonal emergency contraception).

MANIPULATION OF THE MENSTRUAL CYCLE[12]

To postpone a period

Menstrual bleeding can be postponed, short term or longer term as a choice, for the social convenience of women by taking two or more packets of monophasic pills consecutively with no break

This method is not suitable for *phasic preparations*. Women taking two packets of the latter pills consecutively may still bleed, because the first pills from the second packet contain a lower dose of progestogen than the last pills in the first packet. So, women on phasic preparations may delay menstruation, either by continuing to take further tablets from the final phase of another packet of the same brand of the phasic preparation or, alternatively, by transferring directly to a packet of the monophasic brand most similar to the relevant final phase.[12] The original phasic pill can be restarted after the usual seven-day break. Contraceptive efficacy will be maintained throughout.

The tricycle regimen

The tricycle regimen comprises three or four packets of a monophasic pill taken consecutively followed by a break (of four days if the indication is to increase efficacy, otherwise seven days as usual). Women using this longer pill cycle have

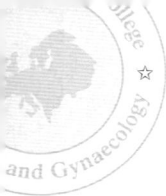

only four or five withdrawal bleeds per year. This regimen is becoming more popular with the introduction of dedicated packaging in some countries (e.g. Seasonale® in the USA, which has 84 active tablets plus seven placebos per pack). But women choosing this option, as they may, should be advised that for any given formulation—as compared with the normal pill cycle—it does increase their annual hormone intake. See Box 2.4.

Postponing uterine bleeding is not always successful. If women experience unacceptable BTB, they should take the pill continuously for a shorter duration (e.g. 'bicycling'), without, if the indication is increased efficacy, changing the planned four-day duration for each PFI.

FOLLOW-UP PROTOCOL[12]

All women should be seen three months after starting the pill (or at one month as appropriate, e.g. in a diabetic or some others with WHO 3 conditions) and then normally every 6–12 months.[28] The acceptability and correct use of the method should be assessed at each visit, any new risk factor should be recorded, and concerns about side effects addressed. The most clinically significant side effects to look out for are a rise in blood pressure and any change in headache pattern (see p. 34). Women should be actively encouraged to return if problems arise, but routine checks should be kept to a minimum and may appropriately be delegated.

Box 2.4 Indications for the tricycle regimen or its variants using a monophasic pill

- At the woman's choice (with advice that, on a four-packs in a row regimen for example, she will consume 16 packs of a given COC per year, not the usual 13)
- Headaches including migraine without aura and other bothersome symptoms occurring regularly in the withdrawal week
- Unacceptably heavy or painful withdrawal bleeds
- Paradoxically, to help women who are concerned about absent withdrawal bleeds—this concern and the nuisance of pregnancy testing therefore arising less often! (Otherwise she may take a triphasic COC in the normal way)
- Endometriosis—for maintenance treatment after primary therapy, a monophasic progestogen-dominant COC may be tricycled
- Pre-menstrual syndrome—tricycling may help, when a COC is used to treat premenstrual syndrome
- Epilepsy—this benefits from relatively more sustained levels of the administered hormone (plus increases efficacy if enzyme-inducing drug is in use; see pp. 41–43).
- Other enzyme-inducer therapy
- Suspicion of decreased efficacy for any other reason

Note: If increased efficacy is required (last three bullets), it is essential also to shorten the PFIs that still occur, usually to four days.

Body weight and BMI. Normally only a baseline measurement of these is useful.

Blood pressure (BP). In contrast, this should be recorded after three months, then every six months into the second year. Thereafter, in all normotensive women without risk factors or relevant disease, WHO strongly endorses a policy of BP measurement being done just annually, with 13 packets of pills issued at a time.[28] However, women with significant risk factors for cardiovascular disease, or who have any chronic medical condition, need more frequent monitoring.

Women who present with symptoms should be investigated and, as indicated, a different pill (see below) or different method may be prescribed.

INDICATIONS FOR STOPPING COC[12]

Any patient who presents with symptoms or signs that indicate a major pill-related side effect should immediately stop taking the pill and take medical advice. Women requesting the pill should be given advance warning (supplemented by a leaflet) of the action they must take if they develop any of the specific symptoms listed in Box 2.5, pending exclusion of a serious cause.

Box 2.5 Reasons to stop the COC—urgently or soon

- Painful swelling in the calf [thrombosis]
- Pleuritic pain in the chest [VTE—this is frequently misdiagnosed as pleurisy]
- Cough with blood-stained sputum or breathlessness [VTE—latter symptom often unrecognised in primary care as due to pulmonary embolism]
- Abdominal pain [abdominal vascular thrombosis, porphyria, gallstones, liver adenoma]
- A bad fainting attack or collapse, or focal epilepsy [stroke]
- Unusual headache; disturbance of speech or visual field, numbness or weakness of a limb especially if asymmetry [distinguish between transient ischaemic attack/incipient stroke—which means urgent neurological referral if suspected—and migraine with focal aura (see p. 34): but stop COC anyway]

Note: The most important possibly pill-related diagnoses are in brackets above. However, in each case there may well be another explanation. Switching to any EE-free (e.g. progestogen-only) method is always appropriate, to maintain contraception.

Discontinuing pill-taking may also be appropriate for some less urgent reasons:

- Sustained hypertension (above 160mmHg systolic or 100mmHg diastolic, or lower in the presence of other risk factors for cardiovascular disease)
- Appearance of a new risk factor(s) or disease constituting an unacceptable risk (e.g. arrival at mid-30s age in a woman who smokes, or age 51 in a healthy non-smoker)
- Onset of jaundice, irrespective of potential cause

> **Box 2.5** Reasons to stop the COC—urgently or soon—(*Continued*)
>
> - Elective surgery—COCs should be stopped four weeks before any surgery known to increase risk of thrombosis (e.g. major surgery or leg surgery, however minor) and restarted at least two weeks after the woman is ambulant; they should also be stopped for four weeks before and four weeks after treatment for varicose veins by surgery or sclerotherapy (injectable or oral progestogens are very suitable for use while the woman is waiting for admission). Major emergency surgery if necessary can be covered by heparin
> - Significant immobilisation of legs, e.g. after fracture
> - Erythema multiforme or other severe skin reaction to COC
> - When pregnancy is desired, or contraception is no longer needed (e.g. post-menopause)

MANAGEMENT OF PROBLEMS AND COMPLICATIONS— BY SYSTEM[5,12]

'MINOR' SIDE EFFECTS[29]

If a change of pill seems appropriate, the main options are:

- a pill with a lower dose of the same progestogen and/or estrogen
- a pill with a different progestogen (usually starting with the lowest available dose)
- a progestogen-only pill.

It is generally not good practice to use other drugs to treat pill-induced side effects. The progestogen-only pill (or another progestogen-only method) may be a satisfactory alternative to the combined pill in women who experience side effects with every brand of COC; however, emotional and psychological factors may contribute to the inability to find an acceptable pill.

CIRCULATORY DISEASES

Hypertension[5]

Hypertension is an important risk factor for heart disease and stroke. Most women on the pill experience a slight increase in systolic and diastolic blood pressure[5] and approximately 1% become clinically hypertensive (incidence increases with age and duration of use). Predisposing factors for pill-induced hypertension include a strong family history and obesity. Pregnancy-induced hypertension does not predispose to hypertension during COC use but a history of this is a risk factor for AMI[8] and hence WHO 2 for the COC method—and WHO 3 in smokers.[27]

Repeated elevated blood-pressure readings are markers of circulatory disease risk, particularly in the presence of other risk factors, such as smoking. According to WHO[27] the combined pill should be stopped in women who have repeated recordings of blood pressure above 160 mmHg systolic or 100 mmHg diastolic. Women with a sustained rise in blood pressure below those levels may be tried with a lower-dose combined pill. If the COC is stopped a progestogen-only preparation is often substituted, and the blood pressure should always be rechecked within three months.

Pill-induced hypertension should not be treated with anti-hypertensive drugs. However, young women with unrelated essential hypertension that is fully controlled by therapy may sometimes (WHO 3) be given a low-dose combined pill, under the supervision of a consultant physician.

Arterial disease
(Including the crucial relevance of any new onset of migraine with aura.)

Venous thromboembolism
(The last two circulatory problems were considered earlier.)

CENTRAL NERVOUS SYSTEM

Depression
Depression used to be a common complaint in women on high-dose pills, but is less common with modern low-dose preparations. Depression appears to be more common in some women who take the pill compared with non-users. However, this may be related to general lifestyle factors rather than to the pill itself.

Some depressed women find the pill very acceptable because it relieves them of one of their greatest fears: unwanted pregnancy. Initial management strategies for depression that might be pill-attributable include lowering the dose of progestogen or changing the progestogen.

Loss of libido
Loss of libido is occasionally reported by women taking the COC, particularly depressed women. This may be linked to psychological problems associated with pill-taking, such as anxiety about its dangers, fears about subsequent fertility or even guilt about using contraception at all. Loss of libido without depression can occur with COCs containing anti-androgens (cyproterone acetate and drospirenone) and is then more likely to improve through a change of brand.

Yet some women actually have increased libido on the COC because the method is reliable, requires no action related to sexual activity, and often reduces premenstrual tension. In all loss of libido cases the family circumstances and psychosexual aspects of the woman's relationship should first be tactfully explored. Remember also that candidiasis may be an indirect cause through vaginal soreness and dryness.

GASTROINTESTINAL SYSTEM

Nausea and vomiting

These are related to the estrogen component of COC and the former should be forewarned about, especially to under-weight women, as a common but transient symptom in the first cycle of pill-taking. Severe vomiting for an unrelated reason may interfere with COC absorption and lead to BTB or spotting.

If nausea or vomiting occur for the first time after months or years of trouble-free pill taking do not forget the possibility of pregnancy!

Pill-related weight gain

This is unusual with all modern COCs, indeed several studies have failed to show any causal link, though it is frequently and unjustifiably expected.

Liver tumours

The relative risk of both benign and malignant primary liver tumours has been reportedly increased by COC use. Fortunately, the background incidence is so small (1–3 per million women per year) that the COC-attributable risk is minimal. No synergism has been found with hepatitis B or C infection; and most reported cases have been in long-term users of relatively high-dose pills that are no longer used.

It is very possible that the association with primary liver cancer may not in fact be a causative one. In a study of mortality rates from this rapidly fatal condition since the 1960s, there was no increase in the USA and Sweden, where OC use has been high, in clear contrast with an increase in Japan, where the COC has been seldom used.[5]

Colorectal cancer

The risk of colorectal cancer appears to be reduced in COC takers, though there are some studies that do not find this protective effect.[5]

GENITAL SYSTEM

Bleeding side effects

Breakthrough bleeding (BTB) or spotting may result from circulating concentrations of steroids that are insufficient to maintain the endometrium, yet it is not usually an indication of an increased risk of pregnancy. BTB is common during the first 2–3 cycles of pill use. Women should be forewarned, and advised to continue taking the pill regularly. Persistent or later BTB should be reassessed/investigated. The invaluable check list in Box 2.6 is modified from one first devised by Sapire.[20]

Absence of withdrawal bleeding is not dangerous, does not signify overdosage, is not related to true secondary 'amenorrhoea' and does not pose any threat to fertility. After excluding pregnancy, the best management is reassurance, or sometimes tricycling (see Box 2.4), or a triphasic pill might be tried.

> **Box 2.6** Checklist for bleeding problems in pill-takers
>
> - Disease—cervical examination; consider chlamydial infection and other cervical causes (polyp, cancer)
> - Disorder of pregnancy—e.g. pill-taking after recent abortion; trophoblastic disease
> - Default—poor compliance
> - Drug-interactions—e.g. recently-initiated enzyme inducers
> - Diarrhoea if *very* severe, and/or vomiting
> - Disturbance of absorption—e.g. after major gut resection
> - Duration—BTB is more common in the first 2–3 months, so persistence with the same product may be rewarded
> - Dose—after the above causes have been excluded, consider a phasic brand or a higher dose product

Cervical cancer

A significant increase of cervical neoplasia in long-term users of COCs compared with controls has now been shown in many studies.[21] Most of these had no accurate information on the sexual activity of the women or their partners. Since the actual carcinogen is transmitted sexually, and a prime candidate is specific strains of the human papilloma virus (HPV), the multi-centre case-control study (referenced in the review[21]) in which all participants were tested for relevant strains of HPV is of particular relevance. In the HPV-positive cervical cancer cases the odds ratios versus controls for use of COCs still increased significantly with greater durations of use.

So the COC is now seen as a co-factor in increasing the likelihood that HPV infection may progress through the pre-invasive stages to invasion. It is probably weaker in this respect than cigarette smoking and, even if the two co-factors are combined, it is believed that routine three-yearly screening by cervical cytology will suffice in ensuring that almost all pre-invasive lesions can be pre-emptively treated. Moreover, past treatment for such lesions is no more than WHO 2 for pill continuation (given ongoing cytological surveillance).

BREAST CANCER

Breast cancer is a common disease, therefore some women will develop it whether or not they take COCs. In the assessment of a possible aetiological link between the pill and breast cancer 'the jury is still out'—despite numerous studies.

The publication by the Collaborative Group on Hormonal Factors in Breast Cancer[7] was based on 90% of available epidemiological data to that date. The Group proposed a model, which is still widely accepted, of an increase in risk through pill usage of 24%—but with diminution in ex-users and complete disappearance of added risk by ten years. The strongest risk factor was confirmed as age of the woman (see Fig 2.3). This is believed to be linked to cumulative exposure of the breast to estrogen/progestogen hormones. The Group found that the most important predictor of added risk with the COC was recency of use.

In 2002, however, a well-conducted major US Centres for Disease Control (CDC) study[17] of 4575 women aged 35–64 with breast cancer and matched controls reported no increased COC-related risk—odds ratios of 1 or less—across the board, for all the following: current users; past users; long-term users; users with a family history; and users starting COCs at a young age. The latter was particularly reassuring, negating the so-called 'time-bomb' for ex-users in this high breast cancer incidence age group, even if exposed before a first full-term pregnancy. This study is very reassuring, given that COC-exposure in the population was >70%, though it is not the 'last word' by any means.

Technically, the upper confidence interval of the overall odds ratio was 1.3. This places the 24% increase in current users that was shown in the 1996 pooled analysis within the bounds, i.e. still maybe corresponding to reality. Moreover, the age range of the CDC study[17] means that it is primarily about breast cancer in ex-users versus controls. It can tell us nothing about those few women (often with genetic predisposition) who get breast cancer under age 35 (not recruited), and little about women who carry on taking the COC from under 35 right through to age 50–51. Very few of the latter were in the studied population, though such long-term use is now permitted as a choice (see below).

In summary, women using COCs can be reassured[12] that:

- If an added breast-cancer risk of the COC exists at all, the highest likely estimate is 24%, and only applies while women are taking the COC and for a few years thereafter; reducing to zero after ten years.
- Beyond ten years after stopping there is no detectable increase in breast cancer risk for former pill users.
- No excess COC-related *mortality* from this cause (or indeed any other cause) has been shown.[3,23]
- The cancers diagnosed in women who use or have ever used COCs are clinically less advanced than those who have never used the pill, and are less likely to have spread beyond the breast.

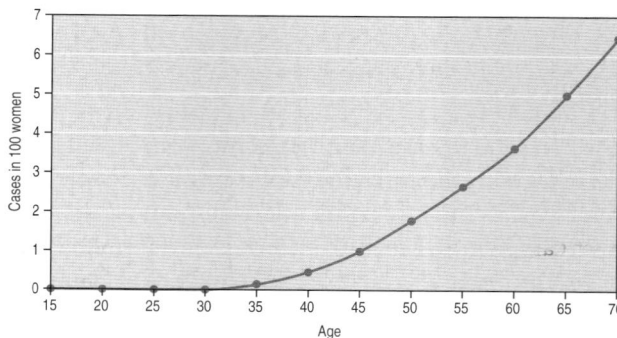

Fig 2.3 Background risk: cumulative number of breast cancers per 100 women, by age. UK data, from Statement by Faculty of Family Planning & Reproductive Healthcare, June 1996. (From Guillebaud 2004,[12] Figure 5.8)

- The risks are not associated with duration of use or the dose or type of hormone in the COC, and there is no synergism with other risk factors for breast cancer (e.g. family history, FH).
- Women who do have a strong FH (breast cancer under age 40, in a sister or mother) do indeed have a pre-existing problem, and if they are known to possess one of the genes BRCA 1 or 2 this would be WHO 4 for the COC. For the larger remainder group with a strong FH, any *added* risk seems the same as for any other woman with no family history. Hence they may certainly use the COC (WHO 2) if they so wish. But they should be advised to request reassessment of their circumstances every five years and earlier as and when new data are obtained.

A good effect of that essentially negative CDC study[17] has been to remove pressure to raise this issue proactively with first-time pill users. The topic should be addressed at an appropriate time, usually in response to questions. Women should be encouraged to practise breast awareness and report any unusual changes promptly. The balancing protective effects of COCs against malignancy of the ovary and endometrium and now, possibly, large bowel are always worth mentioning.

If breast cancer is diagnosed, the prognosis in pill-takers is good. However, the pill should be stopped. It is acceptable (WHO 3) to use progestogen-only methods after prolonged remission, defined by WHO as five years after diagnosis—but always in consultation with the woman's oncologist.

REVERSIBILITY[12]

Irrespective of pill use, women who stop taking COCs generally regain the level of fertility relevant to their age within 1–3 months. The combined pill does not cause any permanent loss of fertility, though the first menstrual period after stopping the pill is often delayed. A few women have amenorrhoea for at least six months, but this is unrelated to the type of pill or duration of use. Secondary amenorrhoea after stopping the pill is not uncommon, particularly in women who have had a late menarche, previous episodes of amenorrhoea or very irregular cycles. Abnormalities that would normally lead to amenorrhoea are masked by regular withdrawal bleeds while on the pill.

Women who fail to menstruate for over six months after stopping the COC should be investigated.

OUTCOME OF PREGNANCY[12]

COC-EXPOSURE PRE-CONCEPTION

Some authorities advise that women should discontinue the pill and use a barrier method of contraception for two to three cycles before a planned conception to enable mineral and vitamin metabolism to normalise. This is not

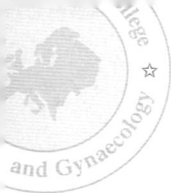

harmful, but there is no objective evidence that it is beneficial. In Europe, the universal use of obstetric diagnostic ultrasound means that accurate identification of the last menstrual period has become less important for calculating gestation. Any woman who becomes pregnant within three months of stopping the pill should be strongly reassured about risk to the baby. After discontinuing the COC, there is no increased risk of miscarriage, ectopic pregnancy or stillbirth, and no alteration in the sex ratio or birth weight. WHO[24] concluded in 1981 that there was no evidence that pill use before conception had any adverse effect on the fetus. No subsequent publications have seriously challenged this view.

EXPOSURE POST-CONCEPTION

Ideally, pregnant women should avoid all drugs, particularly in the first trimester. But a meta-analysis conducted by Bracken in 1990 showed that there was no attributable risk of teratogenesis with COCs (risk ratio 0.99).[6] The incidence of common fetal abnormalities does not seem to be increased in women who take the pill during pregnancy, though there is still some uncertainty about rare abnormalities. The consensus of opinion is that this risk is negligible and therefore therapeutic abortion should not be recommended solely on the basis of the concept of COC-related teratogenesis.

DURATION OF USE AND TAKING BREAKS FROM PILL TAKING[12]

There is no evidence that taking breaks in pill taking enhances fertility or reduces any of the risks. All known risks and benefits associated with the COC apply only during use of the pill, and the risks of long-term use are well balanced by the benefits. Provided pill takers are free of known arterial and venous risk factors, ideally slim, energetic and also migraine-free, COC use may continue to age 50–51 (WHO 3). Yet long-term estrogen-free options like intrauterine devices and systems are usually even better and should always be discussed. Beyond age 51 there are numerous safer means to abolish the tiny residual conception risk.

OTHER COMBINED METHODS

TRANSDERMAL COMBINED HORMONAL CONTRACEPTION: EVRA®

Transdermal combined hormonal contraception (EVRA®, Janssen-Cilag) is an innovative transdermal patch delivering EE with norelgestromin, the active metabolite of NGM (see Fig 2.4). The daily skin dose of 150μg norelgestromin and 20μg EE produces blood levels in the range of those after a tablet of Cilest® but without either diurnal fluctuations or the oral peak dose given to the liver. Pending more specific research information, all the absolute and relative contraindications and indeed most of the above practical management advice about the COC apply, with obvious minor adjustments, to this new product. It appears to be relatively estrogen-dominant, with a bleeding and non-bleeding side-effect

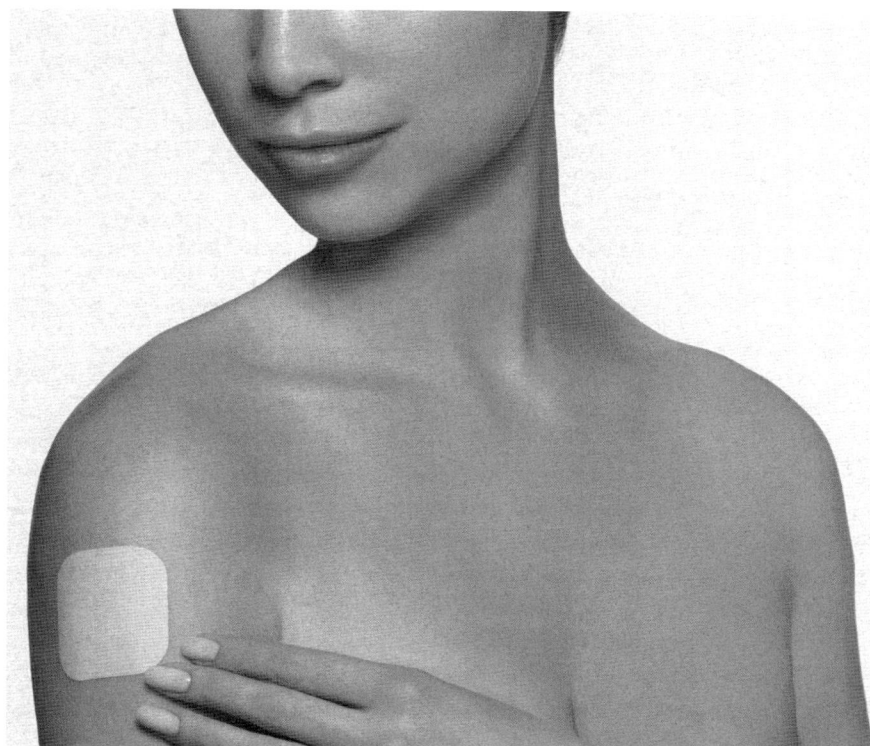

Fig 2.4 The combined contraceptive patch EVRA® applied to the upper arm. (Courtesy of Janssen-Cilag AB)

profile very like Cilest® itself—plus about 2% of women in the trials had local skin reactions that led to discontinuation.

The patch has excellent adhesion, even in hot climates and when bathing or showering. The incidence of detachment of patches was 1.8% (complete) and 2.9% (partial). In the pooled analysis of the RCT studies the Pearl index for consistent users of EVRA® was similar to the oral pills—and less than 1 per 100 woman years.[2] Interestingly, in the clinical trials, one third of the few failures occurred in the 3% weighing above 90 kg. In my view, this apparently reduced effectiveness contraindicates EVRA® for such women who are at least WHO 3 for VTE risk at that level of BMI anyway.

TRANSVAGINAL COMBINED HORMONAL CONTRACEPTION

Already available in some European countries and the USA, NuvaRing® (Organon; see Fig 2.5) is expected in the UK in 2006. It is a combined vaginal ring which releases etonogestrel (3-keto-desogestrel) 120 μg and EE 15 μg per day for 21 days, thus equating to some degree with 'vaginal Mercilon®'. It is normally retained (though there is an option of removing it during sexual activity) for three weeks and then taken out for a withdrawal bleed during the fourth.

Contraception and family planning

Box 2.7 Maintenance of efficacy of EVRA®

- Avoid use at all if body weight is greater than 90 kg

- Each patch is worn for seven days, for three consecutive weeks followed by a patch-free week. This regimen was shown to aid compliance, particularly in young women.[1] Under age 20, perfect use was reported by COC users in 68% of cycles, but in 88% of cycles by patch users. The patch is therefore a useful alternative to offer to those who find it difficult to remember a daily pill, especially as, if the patch user does forget, there is a two-day margin for error for late patch change

  However:

- As with the COC it is essential never to lengthen the contraception-free (patch-free) interval. If this interval exceeds eight days for any reason (either through late application or the first new patch detaching and this being identified late), I advise extra precautions for the duration of the first freshly applied patch (i.e. for seven days). This should be after immediate emergency contraception if there has been sexual exposure during the preceding patch-free time

- There would of course be the possibility of offering it in a 'tricycle' way (as with the COC) meaning the consecutive use of, say, nine or twelve patches before the break. By analogy with the COC this would be more effective for forgetful users and give fewer bleeds, but with more hormone intake per month and at added cost. And since the labelling in the SPC specifies menstrual postponement for just one cycle, this is use of a licensed product in an unlicensed way, so it should be on a 'named patient' basis

- Absorption problems through vomiting/diarrhoea, and tetracycline by mouth, have no effect on this method's efficacy

  But:

- During any short-term enzyme-inducer therapy, and for 28 days after this ends, additional contraception is still advised (as for COCs) plus elimination of any patch-free intervals during this time

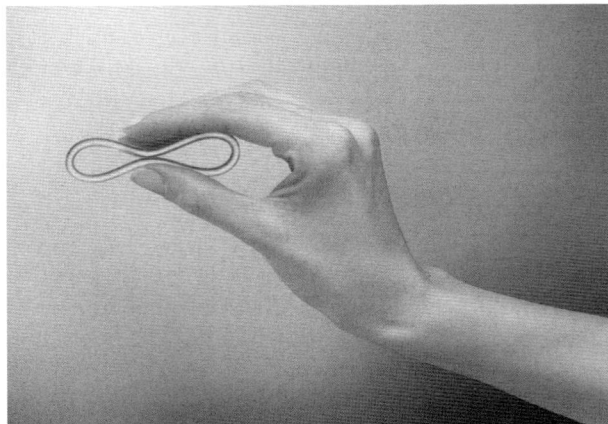

Fig 2.5 NuvaRing®—the contraceptive vaginal ring.
(Courtesy of Organon AB)

Pending more dedicated information, all the absolute and relative contraindications, and most of the above practical management advice about the COC, must be presumed to apply to NuvaRing® (see Box 2.8). It appears to be relatively estrogen dominant, with a side-effect profile very like Mercilon® itself.

In studies at the MPC and elsewhere it proved very popular, with excellent cycle control and once again a failure rate comparable to the COC.[4,19]

CONCLUSIONS

As proposed at the start and now amplified within this chapter, the combined pill is a highly acceptable and reliable method of contraception suitable for most women, and, on balance, it also provides significant *benefits* to their general health during their most fertile years. This advantage is increasingly apparent with respect to both cancer risk and future fertility, yet ironically both are prime areas of anxiety for prospective users who read the popular press!

Although the risks associated with the pill are undeniable and should not be ignored, their incidence is low. So a good way to end is with Fig 2.6, which puts

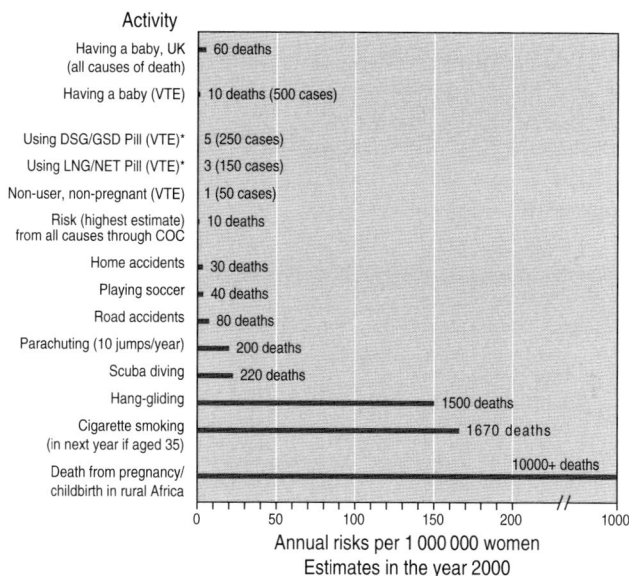

Fig 2.6 The risks of various activities (annual number of deaths per 1 000 000 exposed). With regard to cancer, in this figure excess cancer mortality is assumed to be zero.
COC, combined oral contraceptive; DSG, desogestrel; GSD, gestodene; LNG, levonorgestrel; NET, norethisterone; VTE, venous thromboembolism.
Note: *The extra mortality due to using a DSG/GSD Pill versus a LNG/NET Pill due to VTE equals 2 per million per year. This is equivalent to the average mortality risk from just two hours of driving on UK roads per year (see Practical prescribing, pp. 36–37).
(From Guillebaud 2004,[12] Figure 5.13. Sources: Dinman 1980 Journal of the American Medical Association 244:1226–1228; Mills et al 1996 British Medical Journal 312:121; Anonymous 1991 British Medical Journal 302:743; Strom 1994 Pharmacoepidemiology, 2nd ed, 57–65. Chichester, Wiley; Guillebaud 1998 Contraception today, 3rd ed, 20. London, Martin Dunitz)

Box 2.8 Maintenance of efficacy of NuvaRing®

- Expulsions were a problem for some (usually parous) women, primarily during the emptying of bowels or bladder, and therefore readily recognized

- As with the COC, it will still be essential never to lengthen the contraception-free (ring-free) interval. If for any reason this exceeds eight days, I advise extra precautions for seven days. EC should be added if there has been sexual exposure during any ring-free time of more than eight days

- On the COC model, provided a ring has been intravaginal for a full seven days, after premature expulsion/removal contraceptive efficacy should be restorable just by immediate insertion of a new ring

- There would of course be the possibility of offering it in a tricycle way (as with the COC), meaning the consecutive use of three or four rings before the break

- Absorption problems, vomiting/diarrhoea and broad-spectrum antibiotics have no effect on this method's efficacy

- Additional contraception is still advised with simultaneous enzyme-inducer therapy

them into perspective by comparison with the risks of pregnancy and the normal hazards of day-to-day living.

The provider, doctor or nurse, should always be ready to advise and counsel the woman in a non-directive way while she is on the pill method. To this end they must also ensure that they remain up to date in their knowledge and apply this appropriately to the woman's needs.

References

1. Archer D F, Bigrigg A, Smallwood G H, Shangold G A, Creasy G W, Fisher A C 2002 Assessment of compliance with a weekly contraceptive patch (Ortho Evra/Evra) among North American women. Fertility Sterility 77(2 Suppl 2):S27–S31

2. Audet M C, Moreau M, Koltun W D, Waldbaum A S, Shangold G, Fisher A C, Creasy G W 2001 Evaluation of contraceptive efficacy and cycle control of a transdermal contraceptive patch vs an oral contraceptive. Journal of the American Medical Association 285:2347–2354

3. Beral V, Hermon C, Kay C, Hannaford P, Darby S, Reeves G 1999 Mortality associated with oral contraceptive use: 25 year follow up of cohort of 46 000 women from Royal College of General Practitioners' oral contraception study. British Medical Journal 318:96–100

4. Bjarnadottir R, Tuppurninen M, Killick S R 2002 Comparison of cycle control with a combined contraceptive vaginal ring and oral levonorgestrel/ethinyl estradiol. American Journal of Obstetrics and Gynecology 186:389–395

5. Blackburn R, Cunkelman J, Zlidar V 2000 Oral contraceptives—an update. Population Reports, Series A, No. 9. Baltimore, Population Information Program, 2000:1–39

6. Bracken M 1990 Oral contraception and congenital malformations in offspring: a review and meta-analysis of the prospective studies. Obstetrics and Gynaecology 76:552–557

7. Collaborative Group on Hormonal Factors in Breast Cancer 1996 Breast cancer and hormonal contraceptives: collaborative reanalysis of individual data of 53 297 women with breast cancer and 100 239 women without breast cancer from 54 epidemiological studies. Lancet 347:1713–1727

8. Croft P, Hannaford P C 1989 Risk factors for acute myocardial infarction in women: evidence from the Royal College of General Practitioners' oral contraception study. British Medical Journal 298:165–168

9. Donaghy M, Chang C, Poulter N for the European collaborators of the WHO study of cardiovascular disease and steroid hormone contraception 2002 Duration, frequency, recency, and type of migraine and the risk of ischaemic stroke in women of childbearing age. Journal of Neurology, Neurosurgery and Psychiatry 73:747–750

10. Dunn N, Thorogood M, Faragher B et al 1999 Oral contraceptives and myocardial infarction: results of the MICA case-control study. British Medical Journal 318:1579–1584

11. Guillebaud J 2001 Medical-eligibility criteria for contraceptive use. Lancet 357:1378–1379

12. Guillebaud J 2004 Chapters 5–6: The combined oral contraceptive. In: Guillebaud J Contraception: your questions answered (4th ed). Churchill-Livingstone (Elsevier), Edinburgh, pp 106–272

13. Hamilton C J, Hoogland H J 1989 Longitudinal ultrasonographic study of the ovarian suppressive activity of a low dose triphasic oral contraceptive during correct and incorrect pill intake. American Journal of Obstetrics and Gynecology 161:1159–1162

14. Hannaford P, Webb A 1996 Evidence-guided prescribing of combined oral contraceptives: consensus statement. Contraception 54:125–129

15. Korver T, Goorissen E, Guillebaud J 1995 The combined oral contraceptive pill: what advice should we give when tablets are missed? British Journal of Obstetrics and Gynaecology 102:601–607

16. MacGregor A, Guillebaud J 1998 Recommendations for use of combined oral contraception in women with migraine. British Journal of Family Planning 24:53–60

17. Marchbanks P, McDonald J, Wilson H, Folger S G, Mandel M G, Daling J R et al 2002 Oral contraceptives and the risk of breast cancer. New England Journal of Medicine 346:2025–2032

18. Odlind V, Milsom I, Persson I, Victor A 2002 Can changes in sex hormone binding globulin predict the risk of venous thromboembolism with combined oral contraceptive pills? Acta Obstetricia et Gynecologica Scandinavica 81:482–490

19. Roumen F J M E, Apter D, Mulders T M T, Dieben T O M 2001 Efficacy, tolerability and acceptability of a novel contraceptive vaginal ring releasing etonogestrel and ethinyl estradiol. Human Reproduction 16:469–475

20. Sapire K E (adapted Belfield T, Guillebaud J) 1990 Combined oral contraceptives. Contraception and sexuality in health and disease. McGraw-Hill, London, pp 74–75

21. Smith J, Green J, Berrington de Gonzalez A, Appleby P, Peto J, Plummer M et al 2003 Cervical cancer and use of hormonal contraceptives: a systematic review. Lancet 361:1159–1167

22. Tanis B, van den Bosch M, Kemmeren J, Cats V, Helmerhost F, Algra A et al 2001 Oral contraception and the risk of myocardial infarction. New England Journal of Medicine 345:1787–1793

23. Vessey M, Painter R, Yeates D 2003 Mortality in relation to oral contraceptive use and cigarette smoking. Lancet 362:185–191

24. WHO 1981 The effect of female sex hormones on fetus development and infant health: report of a WHO scientific group. Technical report series 657. WHO, Geneva

25. WHO 1998 Cardiovascular disease and steroid hormone contraception. Report of a WHO Scientific Group. Technical Report Series No. 877. WHO, Geneva

26. WHO 1998 Cardiovascular disease and steroid hormone contraceptives. PROGRESS in Human Reproduction Research 46:1–10

27. WHO/RHR 2004 Medical eligibility criteria for contraceptive use (3rd ed) WHO, Geneva, pp 1–176

28. WHO/RHR 2004 Selected practice recommendations for contraceptive use (2nd ed). WHO, Geneva, pp 1–170

29. Zlidar V 2000 Helping women use the pill. Population Reports, Series A, No. 10. Population Information Program, Baltimore, pp 1–27

3

☆✫☆✫☆✫☆✫☆✫☆✫☆✫☆✫☆✫☆ | ☆

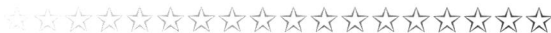

Copper-releasing intrauterine devices

Viveca Odlind

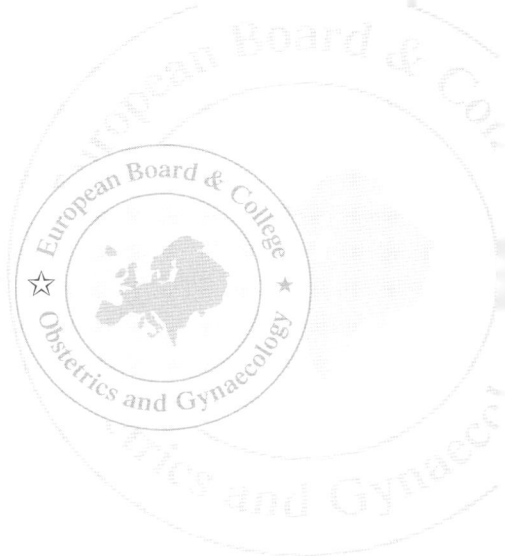

ABSTRACT

Intrauterine device (IUD) use varies between countries from a 30–40% use among fertile women in China to approximately only 1% use in the USA. Acceptability in the USA decreased dramatically as a result of negative publicity related to the Dalkon Shield, which was associated with septic abortions. In the Nordic countries, IUDs are used by 20–25% of fertile women. Early polyethylene IUDs were large and caused much bleeding and pain. Copper IUDs are more effective and cause fewer side effects. The copper surface area is the determinant of contraceptive efficacy. Modern copper IUDs, carrying a higher load of copper, are more effective in preventing pregnancies than earlier IUDs. Most data on the mechanism of action suggest that a copper IUD prevents fertilisation and, thus, is contraceptive and not interceptive. Studies of modern high-load copper IUDs show pregnancy rates close to what is usually found after surgical sterilisation, and some IUDs have a proven lifespan of 10–12 years. The most common reasons for termination are expulsion, bleeding and pain. Termination rates vary between studies and centres, probably also reflecting attitudes among service providers. Varying expulsion rates possibly reflect differences in insertion technique and inserter skill. Older studies suggested an association between IUD use and pelvic inflammatory disease (PID) but more recent studies have not found such an association, except during the first days after insertion. Thus, IUDs are safe for women at low risk of STI, i.e. in mutually monogamous relationships, as sexual behaviour is the most important risk factor for PID. An IUD may therefore be a first choice in most healthy parous women. In an IUD user, a pregnancy is more likely be ectopic, but due to the high contraceptive efficacy of modern IUDs, the absolute numbers of ectopic pregnancies are low. Most studies have shown no harmful effects on subsequent fertility in previous IUD users and no increased risk of tubal infertility in previous nulliparous users of copper IUDs. Because of its high efficacy, long duration, reversibility and low cost, an IUD is one of the most important family-planning methods. Side effects and misconceptions are, however, not uncommon and for high acceptance of the method, careful counselling, medical follow-up and removal facilities should always accompany promotion and use of IUDs.

KEY WORDS

Intrauterine device, copper, Pearl index, pregnancy rate, mechanism of action, menstrual blood loss, pelvic inflammatory disease, nulliparous, return to fertility, ectopic pregnancy

DEVELOPMENT OF INTRAUTERINE CONTRACEPTION

The earliest intrauterine contraceptive devices (IUDs) consisted of a silkworm gut or a metal ring, and were introduced by the German gynaecologist Ernst Gräfenberg in the 1920s. However, those early IUDs never became widely used, presumably because of strong opposition towards the concept of birth control among doctors. It can also be assumed that pelvic infections became a particularly serious medical complication during a time when antibiotics were not yet available. When modern plastic materials, with a 'shape memory' were developed, a renewed interest in intrauterine contraception began. During the late 1950s, the first devices made of polyethylene were developed and IUDs were introduced into family planning programmes in many countries around the world. The early IUD was often coil shaped and was straightened out into a plastic inserter tube and regained its coil shape once it was released from the tube and fitted into the uterine cavity. The early inert IUDs were large and often caused side effects, particularly bleeding and pain.

When intrauterine administration of copper was reported to dramatically reduce the number of implantation sites in rabbits, that discovery resulted in the development of IUDs medicated with copper.[66] Copper IUDs were a great improvement, because not only were they more effective than inert plastic IUDs, with significantly lower pregnancy rates, but they were also smaller and, therefore, caused less bleeding and pain. Most early copper-bearing IUDs were T-shaped and carried a copper surface area of around $200\,mm^2$ copper.

Further clinical research resulted in the development of modern copper IUDs, which carry a higher load of copper than the earlier ones and are significantly more effective in preventing pregnancies than they were. The modern copper IUD that has been most widely studied is the CuT 380A with a total copper surface area of $380A\,mm^2$, which has become the gold standard of modern IUDs. However, several other IUDs with an extended copper surface area have been developed (Fig 3.1). Others are still in clinical trials but may well appear on the market in the near future if they prove equal or superior to the CuT 380A in terms of efficacy, safety, longevity and price. The most recent development of copper IUDs is the frameless device, which consists of copper sleeves on a thread with no plastic frame at all.[33] In an attempt to reduce expulsions as well as bleeding and pain, IUDs releasing hormones, progesterone and subsequently levonorgestrel (Fig 3.1), have been developed (see Ch. 4).

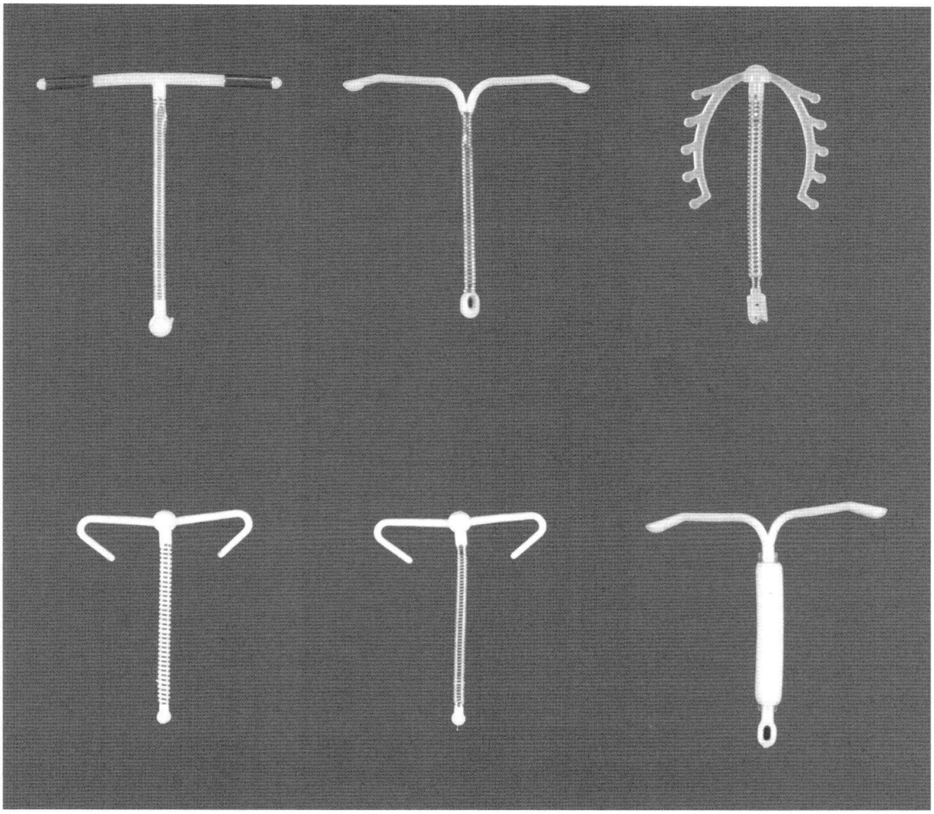

Fig 3.1 Several different types of copper IUD and the levonorgestrel-releasing intrauterine system (IUS) known as Mirena® or Levonova®.
(Courtesy of Professor Ian Milsom)

GLOBAL USE OF COPPER IUDs

Although the concept of intrauterine contraception is widely known throughout the world, the use of IUDs varies considerably between countries, the People's Republic of China being the country in the world where IUDs are most widely used. In the People's Republic of China some 30–40% of women use IUDs, whereas, in the USA, only around 1% of women using contraception use an IUD.[28] In the USA, acceptability of IUD use was initially higher but decreased rapidly and dramatically as a result of negative publicity, most of which was related to the Dalkon Shield, which was reported to be associated with septic spontaneous abortions.[18,50] The Dalkon Shield, in contrast to all current IUDs, had polyfilament tail-strings, which apparently facilitated the ascent of bacteria to the upper genital tract, was withdrawn from the market in the 1970s, but caused almost irreparable damage to the perception of IUD safety in the USA and elsewhere.

IUD use is high in the Nordic countries and in Hungary, whereas relatively few women rely on IUDs in France and the UK.[28] In Sweden, Finland and Norway, IUDs are used by 20–25% of sexually-active fertile women.[34]

IUD DESIGN

Excellent contraceptive efficacy and few side effects and expulsions are obvious prerequisites of an acceptable IUD, but the device also has to be easy to insert and remove. To meet those prerequisites, IUD designers have tried various solutions as can be seen from the numerous varieties of shapes of IUDs. Most modern polyethylene frames are more or less T-shaped with a copper wire on the vertical arm and, in some cases, with copper sleeves on the two horizontal arms. One IUD type does not have a frame at all, but consists of copper sleeves on a thread, which is attached to the uterine fundus by a suture.[33] The copper surface area is an important determinant of the contraceptive efficacy, the larger the surface area, the greater the efficacy.[46] The copper surface area varies in IUDs from $200\,mm^2$ to $380\,mm^2$. Thus, there is evidence for better efficacy in those IUDs with a large copper surface area but there have not been any studies to show whether the location of the copper on the IUD is of importance.

MECHANISM OF ACTION

An IUD in the uterus produces a foreign-body response with a localised trauma in the endometrium, leading to a number of biochemical changes. Those reactions include the appearance of polymorphonuclear leucocytes in the endometrium and in the uterine fluid as well as the invasion of foreign body giant cells, macrophages, plasma cells and mononuclear cells.[42,59] The reaction is enhanced by the release of copper ions and the result is a uterine environment that is toxic to sperms and to the blastocyst.[12,21] Whereas the use of a copper-IUD does not affect ovarian function, there have been studies demonstrating an increased production of prostaglandins in the endometrium, which could simulate uterine and tubal contraction, thereby modifying sperm transport.[32]

Studies attempting to demonstrate whether IUDs are contraceptive or interceptive have looked for the occurrence of embryo-specific substances, i.e. hCG, using sensitive assays. Using a sensitive assay for the detection of hCG, Wilcox et al reported transient occurrence of hCG in only one case out of 109 IUD cycles (0.9%), whereas they found hCG in four cases among 89 control cycles (4.5%). Thus, this study suggested five-times higher rates of fertilisation in the control group compared to the IUD group.[61]

Studies attempting to recover sperms from the tubes of controls and IUD users have reported recovery of a reduced number of sperms from the tubes of IUD users as compared with controls.[12] Ortiz et al, using transcervical flushing of the uterus, found eggs in the uterus in eight out of 36 control non-IUD users, in one out of 22 women with Lippes loop and in none out of 43 women with a CuT 220 IUD.[35] Alvarez et al tried to recover eggs from the fallopian tubes and found no normally developed ova in the fallopian tubes of IUD users compared with controls.[1] Most available data therefore suggest that a copper-releasing IUD in the uterus prevents fertilisation as its main mechanism of action and, thus, acts as a contraceptive.[43]

EFFICACY AND DURATION OF MODERN IUDs

The copper surface area, which has been reported to be the determinant of the contraceptive efficacy, varies in currently used IUDs from 200 mm^2 to 380 A mm^2. There have been several recent large, randomised, comparative studies, showing the excellent efficacy of the modern high-load copper IUDs, i.e. CuT 380 and Multiload 375, with pregnancy rates close to what is usually found after surgical sterilisation (Tables 3.1 and 3.2). In long-term randomised clinical trials the CuT 380A has been found to have significantly lower pregnancy rates than the CuT

Table 3.1 Cumulative discontinuation rates after 36 months. Results from selected randomised comparative studies

Device	Pregnancy	Expulsion	Bleeding/pain	Reference
CuT 220	1.7	4.5	17.3	63
CuT 380A	1.0	7.0	12.9	63
CuT 220	4.4	6.7	11.6	63
Nova-T	6.6	5.8	10.5	63
CuT 220	3.4	7.7	11.9	63
Multiload 250	2.8	3.1	17.6	63
CuT 380Ag	0.6	5.4	8.8	9
Multiload 375	1.8	6.5	11.4	9
CuT 380A	1.6	7.1	7.1	38
FlexiGard (frameless)	2.2	4.1	7.5	38
CuT 380A	0.3	7.38	6.3	64
GyneFix(frameless)	0	3.0	4.5	64
Cu Safe 300	2.5	6.8	10.4	52
CuT 380A	1.5	2.7	15.6	52

Table 3.2 Cumulative discontinuation rates after 60 months. Results from selected randomised comparative studies

Device	Pregnancy	Expulsion	Bleeding/pain	Reference
Nova-T 200	2.2	9.3	26.7	27
CuT 200	5.8	7.2	23.7	27
Nova-T 200	12.3	6.2	15.7	63
CuT 220C	6.6	7.5	15.7	63
CuT 220C	4.0	9.3	17.0	63
CuT 380A	1.4	8.2	18.5	63
Nova-T 200	4.2	5.5	20.4	3
Levonorgestrel IUD	0.3	4.9	15.1	3
CuT 380Ag	1.4	7.4	23.3	45
Levonorgestrel IUD	1.1	11.8	15.4	45

200, the Nova-T and the CuT 220.[10,46,63] The pregnancy rate of the CuT 380 was slightly but not significantly lower than that of the Multiload 250 and the Multiload 375 in other randomised studies.[9,10,11,40,63]

There is now evidence to support the fact that the CuT 380A has an effective lifespan of 10–12 years, during which time the pregnancy rate remains low.[51] Also the Multiload 250 has been shown to remain effective for 8–10 years.[6] The Nova-T had shown an effective lifespan of five years in earlier studies, but in more recent studies the performance of this device, compared with other IUDs, has been shown to deteriorate with prolonged use.[3,27,63] Recent results from a new Nova-T device with an extended copper surface area of 380A mm^2 have demonstrated better efficacy of this device in a non-comparative study over two years as compared with the older prototype.[7] The frameless device, consisting only of copper sleeves, has been shown to have similar efficacy as the CuT 380A in comparative studies over three years.[33,38,64] In summary, several multicentre comparative studies have suggested that the copper IUDs with a high copper load (>300 mm^2) are the most effective, with a cumulative pregnancy rate during five years or more close to 1 per 100 woman years.

REASONS FOR TERMINATION

Side effects occur with IUD use, some of which may lead to discontinuation. The most commonly claimed reasons for termination are expulsion, bleeding and pain (Tables 3.1 and 3.2). Apart from the fact that some IUD users report increase in both dysmenorrhoea and intermenstrual pain, the rates, which vary immensely between studies and centres, probably also reflect variations in attitudes and counselling among service providers. Varying expulsion rates possibly reflect differences in insertion technique and inserter training and skill (Tables 3.1 and 3.2). The frameless IUD types were developed to reduce expulsion rates and terminations for bleeding and pain but in comparative studies so far those IUDs have not been shown to be superior to the CuT 380A.[33]

CHANGE IN MENSTRUAL BLOOD LOSS WITH COPPER IUDs

INCREASED MENSTRUAL BLOOD LOSS

All inert and copper-releasing IUDs increase menstrual blood loss (MBL). Although some studies suggest that the volume of MBL is highest during the first cycles after insertion, most investigations suggest that most of the increase in MBL will remain throughout the whole period of IUD use.[5,39] The magnitude of the increase in MBL is related to the size of the device. With larger types of IUDs, i.e. Lippes loop and other plastic non-medicated devices, MBL has been shown to increase by at least 100%.[41] Smaller copper devices, i.e. CuT 200, Nova-T, CuT 380A and Multiload, generally cause an increase in MBL by 40–80%.[5,31] Although assessments of MBL and termination rates for bleeding vary considerably between studies, there is little evidence for a real difference between different copper IUDs in general. One study demonstrated no difference in MBL, when comparing Multiload 375 and Multiload 250, suggesting that the amount of copper release does not affect MBL.[29]

The mechanism for the increased MBL is not fully understood. The trauma and foreign-body reaction in the endometrium adjacent to the device will result in increased vascularity as well as a local increase in fibrinolytic activity.[39,42] IUD users have also been reported to have increased endometrial plasminogen activator concentrations as well as superficial endometrial erosions, leading to microvascular bleeding into the cavity and increased vascular permeability, leading to interstitial haemorrhage.[24,42] Another factor contributing to the increased blood loss may be alterations in the balance between prostaglandins, mainly prostacyclin (which inhibits haemostasis through vasodilatation and prevents platelet aggregation) and thromboxane A2, which has the opposite effect.[42,48] More recent data have also suggested increased lysosomal enzyme activity in the endometrium of IUD users as contributing to the increased MBL.[58]

PROLONGED MENSTRUAL BLEEDING

Users of inert or copper IUDs often report a prolongation of their menstrual period by 1–2 days. In some studies this type of bleeding is referred to as intermenstrual spotting, but is more likely directly related to the endocrine menstrual cycle changes. It has been demonstrated that in IUD users the menstrual bleeding starts before progesterone levels have decreased to the low levels at which the normal menstruation is usually precipitated.[32] The mechanism behind this premature precipitation of menstruation, resulting in prolongation of the menstruation, in IUD users is supposedly related to the localised trauma in the endometrium. Use of a copper IUD does not affect ovarian function.[32]

INTERMENSTRUAL BLEEDING

Many IUD users report 1–3 days of spotting during the midcycle, a sign which may be explained by a drop in estrogen levels subsequent to ovulation, precipitating bleeding in a predisposed endometrium. There are no recent studies to confirm whether this explanation is valid or not. The blood volume lost at intermenstrual bleeding is usually insignificant for the health of the woman but may affect acceptability and considerably reduce continuation of the method.[41] Intermenstrual bleeding in IUD users, particularly bleeding occurring at random during the cycle, should be considered as potentially pathological until properly evaluated since it may be a symptom of an underlying pathology, which is unrelated to IUD use, i.e. infection or neoplasia.

HEALTH IMPACT OF INCREASED MBL

The amount of blood loss at normal menstruation without IUD varies between populations. The MBL in healthy women is often reported to be around 40 ml and

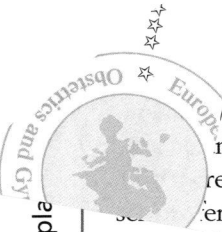

.ore in certain Asian countries, i.e. the People's Republic of China and
With an MBL of 60–80 ml or more, most women will develop a negative
nce, a depletion of iron stores and subsequently iron deficiency anaemia.
rease in MBL subsequent to IUD insertion is reflected in a reduction of
erritin levels.[5,39] The haemoglobin level is a less accurate early marker of
increased MBL in IUD users, but haemoglobin levels will decrease if excessive MBL
is allowed to continue. The health consequences even of a moderately increased
MBL may be severe in women with pre-existing anaemia and/or low iron intake.[39]

MANAGEMENT OF BLEEDING DISTURBANCES DURING COPPER IUD USE

Perception of MBL is very subjective and it is often difficult to obtain an adequate assessment of the volume of MBL by patient history.[17] Treatment with antifibrinolytic drugs, i.e. tranexamic acid, will reduce MBL by around 50%.[30] Mefenamic acid and other NSAIDs will reduce MBL by around 25%.[26,65] Therefore, such drugs can usually control a moderate increase in MBL in otherwise healthy women and IUD use could continue. Removal should, however, be recommended if treatment with antifibrinolytic drugs or NSAIDs does not reduce the MBL. IUD removal should be considered in all cases of intolerable bleeding and/or anaemia, or if there is a suspicion of underlying pathology.

Women who cannot tolerate the prolongation of the bleeding period by 1–2 days or a short episode of midcycle intermenstrual spotting should be advised to have the IUD removed, since this is usually not possible to treat.

PELVIC INFLAMMATORY DISEASE

Although evidence of a direct association between previous IUD use and infertility is scarce, several case-control studies performed in the past suggested a strong association between IUD use and the risk of PID.[18,53,60] Subsequent reanalyses of older studies have pointed at several possible biases, in particular the choice of control group, which may have had benefit from the protective effect of other contraceptive methods.[8,19,25] The potential for misclassification bias as a possible association between PID and IUD use had been postulated, making the diagnosis PID more likely to have been made in IUD users. In the selection of candidates for IUD use in the past, such issues as possible existing risk factors for sexually transmitted infections (STIs) in the woman and/or her male partner may have been overlooked. Reanalysis of older studies and a more recent study from WHO have not been able to demonstrate any substantial risk increase for PID among IUD users, provided that a careful pre-insertion counselling and patient evaluation was made, except during the first 20 days after insertion, a risk attributed to the transfer of bacteria into the uterus at the time of IUD insertion.[15,19] It now seems clear that IUDs offer no protection against STIs but are safe for women in mutually monogamous relationships. A cohort study of HIV-infected women using copper IUDs did not suggest increase in complications or viral shedding.[19]

Thus, most results suggest that sexual behaviour is the most important risk factor for PID, but it has not been possible to separate the influence of age and parity on PID risk in IUD users from sexual behaviour. In the WHO study, nulliparous women were not included and there was an inverse correlation between PID and age. Therefore, whereas IUD may well be a first choice in parous women, it is still a second option in young, nulliparous women.

In a recent case-control study of women over 25, presenting with clinical PID, IUD use was not associated with PID in general, but IUD users >35 had an increased risk of PID. The study suggested that the possible pathogenesis of PID was a synergistic effect between several anaerobic and aerobic pathogens, possibly facilitated by the presence of an IUD.[56]

ECTOPIC PREGNANCY

The risk of ectopic pregnancy is strongly related to the total risk of pregnancy associated with an IUD. Early studies suggested that IUD users had higher than expected rates of ectopic pregnancies and that the ectopic rate seemed to increase with prolonged duration of IUD use.[14,55] In a subsequent reanalysis of their data, Vessey et al found that ectopic pregnancy rates did not significantly increase with duration of IUD use.[55] More recent prospective studies of highly effective IUDs failed to demonstrate any negative effect of duration on risk and showed rates of ectopic pregnancy among IUD users that were similar to those of users of other highly effective contraceptive methods.[44] In a review, Sivin pointed out that the absolute rate of ectopic pregnancy is extremely low with the most effective IUDs because of the low total pregnancy rate with those devices (Table 3.3). Thus, whereas the ratio between ectopic and intrauterine pregnancy in IUD users is increased as compared with non-contracepting women, the absolute numbers are low and therefore it can be concluded that use of modern IUDs is protective against ectopic pregnancy.[44]

NULLIPARITY AND IUD USE AND RETURN OF FERTILITY

There have been both cohort and case-control studies, showing no harmful effects on subsequent fertility in previous IUD users.[2,36,47,54] Recently, Hubacher

Table 3.3 Rate of ectopic pregnancy during the first two years of randomised trials of non-medicated IUDs (Lippes loop), copper-releasing IUDs with copper area of 200 mm^2 or less, copper-releasing IUDs with copper area of more than 200 mm^2, and during five years with the Levonorgestrel-releasing IUD

Type of device	Woman years	Pregnancies per 1000	Per cent ectopic	Ectopics per 1000
Non-medicated	4600	19.0	4.6	0.87
Cu < 200 mm^2	21200	20.8	3.6	0.75
Cu > 200 mm^2	39200	7.3	3.2	0.23
Levonorgestrel IUD	5600	0.9	20.0	0.20

(Adapted from Sivin[45])

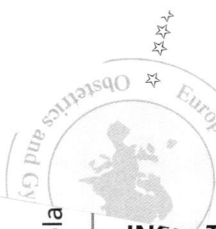

orted no increased risk of tubal infertility in previous nulliparous users
r IUDs whereas Doll et al[13] found an impairment in fertility associated
.g-term IUD use in nulliparous women.

INSERTION AND FOLLOW-UP

The most effective available IUD, in terms of pregnancy protection, should
always be recommended. It is also important that the selected IUD is easy to
insert and remove and that it has a reasonably long duration of proven efficacy,
since the greatest risk of complication occurs in connection with insertion. It is
also important that anyone who inserts IUDs has adequate gynaecological training for this procedure.

TIMING OF IUD INSERTION

An IUD can be inserted at any time during the menstrual cycle when it is reasonable to believe that the woman is not pregnant. Insertion can safely be done
immediately post-abortion in the first trimester if no infection is suspected.[49] A
copper IUD can also be inserted immediately postpartum within 48 hours after
delivery, although expulsion rates are usually higher at that time.[20] IUD insertion
during lactational amenorrhea is also safe but can be associated with an increased
risk of unnoticed uterine perforation, presumably because of the thin and small
size of the uterus in that endocrine situation.[4] There are no increases in serum
ceruloplasmin or copper concentrations in breast milk in breastfeeding women
fitted with a copper IUD.[37]

PRE-INSERTION EVALUATION

Before IUD insertion, a history should be obtained, including parity, last menstrual period, previous medical history, STI screening by history. The woman
should be carefully counselled about efficacy, mechanism of action, possible side
effects, including the effects on menses, and other possible risks. Finally, a specu-
lum and bimanual pelvic examination should be done. Laboratory tests are not
mandatory for IUD use, but, according to local routines, haemoglobin, pregnancy
test, wet smear, and cervical cancer screening may be appropriate. There is no
evidence for any beneficial effect of routine use of prophylactic antibiotics in
connection to IUD insertion.[57]

FOLLOW-UP ROUTINES

One follow-up visit after 3–6 weeks, around the time of highest incidence of
post-insertion infection, could be recommended for additional counselling and
support. Subsequent visits are encouraged for perceived problems but routine
check-up visits do not usually contribute to user satisfaction. During recent years,
use of ultrasonography (US) has sometimes become part of the assessment

procedure of IUD performance. In a recent study, however, Faundes et al pointed out that there is no correlation between common complaints, such as bleeding and pain, and intrauterine IUD position as assessed by US.[16] Therefore, it seems reasonable to suggest that decisions regarding management of perceived IUD-related problems should rely primarily on clinical evaluation.

CONCLUSION

Given the new understanding of IUDs, both the mode of contraceptive action, the high efficacy and lack of association with PID and infertility and the fact that most IUDs are inexpensive, resulting in a favourable cost-benefit ratio, it seems reasonable and likely that IUD use should increase in the future. A recent systematic review of IUD data reported several non-contraceptive benefits of IUD use, one being the reduced incidence of endometrial cancer reported among IUD users.[23]

Whilst intrauterine contraception is one of the most important long-term family planning methods, menstrual bleeding disturbance remains a common problem and a factor that can limit method acceptability among women in all societies. Therefore, from a reproductive health perspective, it is important that careful counselling, medical follow-up and removal facilities always accompany promotion and use of intrauterine contraceptive methods.

References

1. Alvarez F, Brache V, Fernandez E et al 1988 New insights on the mode of action of intrauterine contraceptive devices in women. Fertility and Sterility 49:768–773
2. Andersson K, Batar I, Rybo G 1992 Return to fertility after removal of a levonorgestrel-releasing intrauterine device and Nova-T. Contraception 46:575–584
3. Andersson K, Odlind V, Rybo G 1994 Levonorgestrel-releasing and copper-releasing (Nova-T) IUDs during five years of use. Contraception 49:56–72
4. Andersson K, Ryde-Blomqvist E, Lindell K, Odlind V, Milsom I 1998 Perforations with intrauterine devices: report from a Swedish survey. Contraception 57:251–255
5. Andrade A T L, Orchard E P 1987 Quantitative studies on menstrual blood flow in IUD users. Contraception 36:129–144
6. Batar I 1985 ML Cu 250 IUD: a decade of experience. Advances in Contraception 1:329–335
7. Batar I, Kuukankorpi A, Rauramo I, Siljander M 1999 Two-year clinical experience with Nova-T 380, a novel copper–silver IUD. Advances in Contraception 15:37–48

8. Buchan H, Villard-Mackintosh L, Vessey M, Yeates D, McPherson K 1990 Epidemiology of pelvic inflammatory disease in parous women with special reference to intrauterine device use. British Journal of Obstetrics and Gynaecology 97:780–788
9. Champion C B, Behlilovic B, Arosemena J M, Randic L, Cole L P, Wilkens L R 1988 A three-year evaluation of the CuT 380Ag and Multiload 375 intrauterine device. Contraception 38:631–639
10. Chi I C, Farr G, Thompson K, Acosta M, Alvarado G, Rivera R, Bandaragoda J, Betancourt J D 1990 Is the copper T 380A device associated with increased risk of removal due to bleeding and pain? An analysis. Contraception 42:159–169
11. Cole L P, Potts D M, Aranda C, Behlilovic B, Etman E S, Moreno J, Randic L 1985 An evaluation of the CuT 380Ag and the Multiload Cu 375. Fertility and Sterility 43:214–217
12. Croxatto H B, Ortiz M E, Valdez E 1994 IUD mechanisms of action. In: Bardin C W, Mishell D R Jr (eds) Proceedings from the Fourth International Conference on IUDs. Butterworth-Heinemann, Boston, pp 44–62

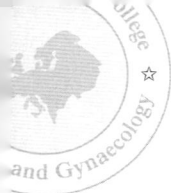

13. Doll H, Vessey M, Painter R 2001 Return of fertility in nulliparous women after discontinuation of the intrauterine device: comparison with women discontinuing other methods of contraception. British Journal of Obstetrics and Gynaecology 108:304–314

14. Edelman D A, Porter C W 1987 The intrauterine device and ectopic pregnancy. Contraception 36:85–96

15. Farley T M, Rosenberg M J, Rowe P J, Chen J H, Meirik O 1992 Intrauterine devices and pelvic inflammatory disease: an international perspective. Lancet 339:785–788

16. Faundes D, Bahamondes L, Faundes A, Petta C, Diaz J, Marchi N 1997 No relationship between the IUD position evaluated by ultrasound and complaints of bleeding and pain. Contraception 56:43–47

17. Fraser I S, McCarron G, Markham R 1984 A preliminary study of factors influencing perceptions of menstrual blood loss volume. American Journal of Obstetrics and Gynecology 149:788–793

18. Gareen I F, Greenland S, Morgenstern H 2000 Intrauterine devices and pelvic inflammatory disease: meta-analysis of published studies, 1974–1990. Epidemiology 11:589–597

19. Grimes D 2000 Intrauterine device and upper genital tract infection. Lancet 356:1013–1019

20. Grimes D, Schulz K, van Vliet H, Stanwood N 2002 Immediate postpartum insertion of intrauterine devices: a Cochrane Review. Human Reproduction 17:549–554

21. Holland M K, White I G 1988 Heavy metals and human spermatozoa. III The toxicity of copper ions for spermatozoa. Contraception 38:685–695

22. Hubacher D, Lara-Ricalde R, Taylor D J, Guerra-Infante F, Guzman-Rodriguez R 2001 Use of copper intrauterine device and the risk of tubal infertility among nulligravid women. New England Journal of Medicine 345:561–567

23. Hubacher D, Grimes D 2002 Noncontraceptive benefits of intrauterine devices: a systematic review. Obstetrical Gynecological Survey 57:120–128

24. Kasonde J M, Bonnar J 1976 Aminocaproic acid and menstrual blood loss in women using intrauterine devices. British Medical Journal 4:17–19

25. Kronmal R A, Whitney C W, Mumford S D 1991 The intrauterine device and pelvic inflammatory disease: The Women's Health Study reanalysed. Journal of Clinical Epidemiology 44:109–122

26. Lethaby A, Augood C, Duckitt K 2002 Non-steroidal anti-inflammatory drugs for heavy menstrual bleeding (Cochrane Review). In The Cochrane Library 4. Update Software, Oxford

27. Luukkainen T, Allonen H, Nielsen N C, Nygren K G, Pyörälä T 1983 Five years' experience of intrauterine contraception with the Nova-T and the Copper T 200. American Journal of Obstetrics and Gynecology 147:885–892

28. Mauldin W P, Segal S J 1994 IUD use throughout the world: past, present and future. In Bardin CW, Mishell D R Jr (eds) Proceedings from the Fourth International Conference on IUDs. Butterworth-Heinemann, Guildford, pp 1–10

29. Milsom I, Rybo G, Lindstedt G 1989 The influence of copper surface area on menstrual blood loss and iron status in women fitted with an IUD. Contraception 41:271–281

30. Milsom I, Andersson K, Andersch B, Rybo G 1991 A comparison of flurbiprofen, tranexamic acid, and a levonorgestrel-releasing intrauterine contraceptive device in the treatment of idiopathic menorrhagia. American Journal of Obstetrics and Gynecology 164:879–883

31. Milsom I, Andersson K, Jonasson K, Lindstedt G, Rybo G 1995 The influence of the Gyne T 380S IUD on menstrual blood loss and iron status. Contraception 52:175–179

32. Nygren K G, Johansson E D B 1973 Premature onset of menstrual bleeding during ovulatory cycles in women with an intrauterine contraceptive device. American Journal of Obstetrics and Gynecology 117:971–975

33. O'Brian P A, Marfleet C 2002 Frameless versus classical intrauterine device for contraception. (Cochrane Review) The Cochrane Library, Issue 4. Update software, Oxford

34. Oddens B, Milsom I 1996 Contraceptive practice and attitudes in Sweden 1994. Acta Obstetricia et Gynecologica Scandinavica 75:932–940

35. Ortiz M E, Croxatto H B, Bardin C W 1996 Mechanism of action of intrauterine devices. Obstetrical Gynecological Survey 51(Suppl):42–51

36. Pyorala T, Allonen H, Nygren K G, Nielsen N C, Luukkainen T 1982 Return of fertility

after the removal of Nova-T or copper T 200. Contraception 26:113–120

37. Rodrigues da Cunha A C, Dorea J G, Cantuaria A A 2001 Intrauterine device and maternal copper metabolism during lactation. Contraception 63:37–39

38. Rowe P J, Reinprayoon D, Koetsawang S, Shu-rong Z, Shang-zun W, Hui-min F et al 1995 The CuT 380A IUD and the frameless IUD 'the Flexigard': interim three-year data from an international multicentre trial. Contraception 52(2):77–83

39. Rybo G, Andersson K 1994 IUD use and endometrial bleedings. In: Bardin C W, Mishell D R Jr (eds) Proceedings from the Fourth International Conference on IUDs. Butterworth-Heinemann, Guildford, pp 210–218

40. Sastrawinata S, Farr G, Prihadi S M, Hutapea H, Anwar M, Wahyudi I, Sunjoto M D, Kemara P, Champion C B, Robbins M 1991 A comparative clinical trial of the CuT 380A, Lippes' loop D, and Multiload Cu 375 IUDs in Indonesia. Contraception 44:141–154

41. Shaw S T, Andrade A T L, Souza J P, Macauley L K, Rowe P J 1980 Quantitative menstrual and intermenstrual blood loss in women using Lippes' loop and copper T intrauterine devices. Contraception 21:343–352

42. Sheppard B L 1987 Endometrial morphological changes in IUD users. A review. Contraception 36:1–10

43. Sivin I 1989 IUDs are contraceptives, not abortifacients: a comment on research and belief. Studies Family Planning 20:355–359

44. Sivin I 1991 Dose- and age-dependent ectopic pregnancy risks with intrauterine contraception. Obstetrics and Gynecology 78:291–298

45. Sivin I, El Mahgoub S, McCarthy T, Mishell D R Jr, Shoupe D, Alvarez F, Brache V, Jimenez E, Diaz J, Faundes A, Diaz M, Coutinho E, Mattos C E, Diaz S, Pavez M, Stern J 1990 Long-term contraception with the levonorgestrel 20 mcg/day (LNg 20) and the Copper T 380Ag intrauterine devices: a five-year randomised study. Contraception 42:361–378

46. Sivin I, Stern J 1979 Long-acting, more effective copper IUDs: a summary of US experience. Studies Family Planning 10: 263–281

47. Skjeldestad F, Bratt H 1988 Fertility after complicated and non-complicated use of IUDs: a controlled perspective study. Advances in Contraception 4:179–184

48. Smith S K, Abel M H, Kelly R W, Baird D T 1981 Prostaglandin synthesis in the endometrium of women with ovular dysfunctional uterine bleeding. British Journal of Obstetrics and Gynaecology 88:434–442

49. Stanwood N L, Grimes D A, Schulz K F 2001 Insertion of an intrauterine contraceptive device after induced or spontaneous abortion. British Journal of Obstetrics and Gynaecology 108:1168–1173

50. Tatum H J, Schmidt F H, Phillips D, McCarty M, O'Leary W M 1975 The Dalkon Shield controversy. Structural and bacteriological studies of IUD tails. Journal of the American Medical Association 231:711–717

51. United Nations Development programme/United Nations Population Fund/World Health Organization/World Bank/Special Programme of Research, Development and Research Training in Human Reproduction 1997 Long-term reversible contraception: twelve years of experience with the CuT 380A and CuT 220C. Contraception 56:341–352

52. Van Kets H E, Van der Pas H, Delbarge W, Thiery M 1995 A randomised comparative study of the CuT 380A and Cu-Safe 300 IUDs. Advances in Contraception 11:123–129

53. Vessey M P, Yeates D, Flavel R, McPherson K 1981 Pelvic inflammatory disease and the intrauterine device: findings in a large cohort study. British Medical Journal 282:855–857

54. Vessey M P, Lawless M, McPherson K, Yeates D 1983 Fertility after stopping use of intrauterine contraceptive device. British Medical Journal 286:106

55. Vessey M P, Yeates D, Flavel R 1979 Risk of ectopic pregnancy and duration of use of an intrauterine device. Lancet 8:501–502

56. Viberga I, Odlind V, Lazdane G, Kroica J, Berglund L, Olofsson S 2004 Microbiology profile in women with pelvic inflammatory disease in relation to IUD use. Infectious Diseases Obstetrics Gynecology (in press)

57. Walsh T, Grimes D, Frezieres R et al 1998 Randomised controlled trial of prophylactic antibiotics before insertion of intrauterine devices. Lancet 351:1005–1008

58. Wang I Y, Fraser I S, Barsamian S P, Manconi F, Street D J, Cornillie F J, Russell P 2000 Endometrial lysosomal activity in ovulatory dysfunctional bleeding, IUCD users and postpartum women. Molecular Human Reproduction 6:258–263

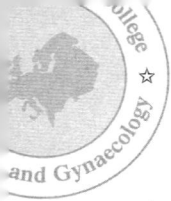

59. Wang I Y, Russell P, Fraser I S 1995 Endometrial morphometry in users of intrauterine contraceptive devices and women with ovulatory dysfunctional bleeding: a comparison with normal endometrium. Contraception 51:243–248

60. Weström L 1975 Effect of acute pelvic inflammatory disease on fertility. American Journal of Obstetrics and Gynecology 121:707–713

61. Wilcox A J, Weinberg C R, Armstrong E G, Canfield R E 1987 Urinary human chorionic gonadotropin among intrauterine device users: detection with highly specific and sensitive assay. Fertility and Sterility 47:265–269

62. World Health Organization 1987 Mechanism of action, safety and efficacy of intrauterine devices. Technical Report Series 753

63. World Health Organisation 1990 The CuT 380A, CuT 220C, Multiload 250 and Nova-T IUDs at three, five and seven years of use—results from three randomised multicentre trials. Contraception 42:141–158

64. Wu S, Hu J, Wildemeersch D 2000 Performance of the frameless Gynefix and the CuT 380A IUDs in a three-year multicentre, randomised, comparative trial in parous women. Contraception 61(2):91–98

65. Ylikorkala O, Viinikka L 1983 Comparison between antifibrinolytic and antiprostaglandin treatment in the reduction of increased menstrual blood loss in women with intrauterine contraceptive device. British Journal of Obstetrics and Gynaecology 90:78–83

66. Zipper J A, Medel M and Prager R 1969 Experimental suppression of fertility by intrauterine copper and zinc in rabbits. American Journal of Obstetrics and Gynecology 105:529–534

4

☆☆☆☆☆☆☆☆☆☆☆☆☆☆☆☆☆☆☆☆ ☆

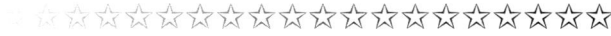

Medicated IUDs

Carl Gustaf Nilsson

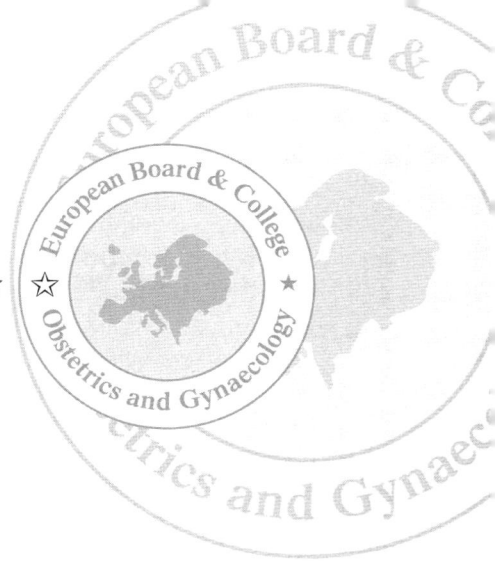

ABSTRACT

The idea of adding a bioactive agent to an intrauterine device in order to overcome some of the problems associated with the clinical use of intrauterine contraceptive devices was tested in animal models during the 1960s. By the beginning of the 1970s clinical trials had been initiated. In the search for the most suitable hormone to be added to the devices, the synthetic progestin levonorgestrel, was found to have the most favourable features. A levonorgestrel-releasing intrauterine system has been most widely evaluated and has led to the commercial introduction of Mirena® or Levonova® for contraceptive use. Mirena® is a highly effective, long-acting and rapidly reversible method of contraception, which offers additional health benefits and therapeutic possibilities through its strong suppressive effect on the endometrium.

KEYWORDS

Contraception, intrauterine, progestins, levonorgestrel, mode of action, health benefit

INTRODUCTION

All intrauterine devices (IUDs) that release any kind of bioactive substances can be regarded as medicated. Although the most widely used IUDs presently are the copper-releasing models, this chapter will deal only with intrauterine hormone-releasing systems. A separate chapter on copper-releasing IUDs is presented elsewhere in this volume (see Ch. 3).

During the 1960s intrauterine devices became an important method of contraception. Although the main reasons for discontinuation of use were bleeding and pain, one of the disadvantages of this method was the high percentage of expulsion. The expulsion rates for certain IUDs tended to rise above 20%.

At the same time the combined oral contraceptive pill (COC) was recognised as the most effective reversible method. However, as experience with COCs increased, the majority of side effects were attributed to the estrogen component. In addition, a weakness of the oral contraceptive method is that effectiveness is dependant on daily motivation to take the pill. Since the demonstration, in 1965, of the contraceptive efficacy of estrogen-free low-dose progestins,[24] investigations have been undertaken into various modes of administrations of progestins for contraceptive purposes.

On the assumption that local intrauterine administration of a progestin would decrease uterine sensitivity and contractility and thus enhance retention of intrauterine devices Doyle and Clewe[7] studied the effect of hormone-releasing intrauterine devices on the rate of expulsion in rats and rabbits. This was the first report on intrauterine administration of a progestin by sustained release and demonstrated that sufficiently high concentrations of progestins completely prevented expulsion. Later it was shown that intrauterine progesterone had an antifertility effect in the rabbit.

In the early 1970s several parallel clinical trials with intrauterine administration of different progestins by means of various devices were initiated. The progestins tested were medroxyprogesterone acetate, crystalline progesterone, norethisterone and d-norgestrel. The clinical results with different shapes of silastic intrauterine devices containing medroxyprogesterone acetate were poor. Intrauterine systems releasing progesterone reached the stage of being marketed under the trade name of Progestasert®. This IUD released 65 µg of crystalline progesterone daily and had an effective lifetime of initially one year and later a lifetime of two years when the amount of progesterone contained in the IUD was increased from 38 mg to 52 mg. In randomised studies comparing Progestasert® with widely used copper-releasing IUDs the termination rates because of bleeding problems were significantly higher with Progestasert®. The same reports also showed a significantly higher pregnancy rate in Progestasert® users.[34] The unacceptably high rates of ectopic pregnancy were also of great concern and finally resulted in withdrawal of Progestasert® from the market in all but two countries. In a small trial with a norethisterone-releasing device a relatively steady release of the steroid from a silastic rod was achieved, but broad peaks of endogenous estradiol during ovulatory cycles and a calculated short life-span of the device were reasons for not developing this concept further.[13]

LEVONORGESTREL-RELEASING INTRAUTERINE SYSTEM (LNG-IUS)

D-norgestrel, which is better known as levonorgestrel, became the steroid that was most suitable for intrauterine administration and had the most advantageous release properties. It was not just by chance that levonorgestrel was chosen. The prerequisites for a long-lasting constant intrauterine release of a steroid are (a) high potency on a per weight basis and (b) slow diffusion through the carrier material.

Among the synthetic progestins available in the early 1970s levonorgestrel was not only the most potent progestin but was also regarded as safe on the basis of clinical experience. When the release properties of progesterone, medroxyprogesterone acetate, norgestrel and chlormadinone acetate were compared those of norgestrel were found to be the slowest.

Due to uneven hydrolysis of the polylactate material in utero, the first clinical trial with levonorgestrel contained in a polylactate material did not result in the desired release of the hormone. The use of silicon, a polydimethylsiloxane polymer, as the carrier material for levonorgestrel resulted in fairly constant release rates. It was found possible to regulate the release rate by variation of both the physical properties and the surface area of the silicon carrier.[16] Radioimmunoassay determinations of plasma concentrations of levonorgestrel and sex hormones showed that the intrauterine release rate was reflected in plasma levels of levonorgestrel and in the effect on ovulatory function. To meet the requirements of long-acting contraception the release rate chosen was 20 μg per day. Release rates between 10 and 100 μg had been tested, but 20 μg per day had the most favourable clinical performance. The first large comparative field study to compare a levonorgestrel-releasing intrauterine system with a copper-releasing IUD showed that the 20 μg releasing system was more effective in preventing pregnancy than the copper-releasing device.[17]

MECHANISM OF ACTION OF THE LEVONORGESTREL-RELEASING INTRAUTERINE SYSTEM

EFFECT ON THE ENDOMETRIUM

Although the LNG-IUS is a hormonal contraceptive method, the mechanism by which it exerts its contraceptive effect is distinctly different from that of the oral contraceptives and IUDs.

The effect on the endometrium is the most profound and most important. There is a uniform suppression of endometrial proliferation regardless of the phase of the menstrual cycle, the duration of use or the age or parity of the user.[29] The histological appearance of the endometrium is one of inactivity, with a thin epithelium and a decidualisation of the stroma. The foreign-body reaction usually seen during IUD use is weaker during use of the LNG-IUS. These changes are the result of the high local concentrations of levonorgestrel in the endometrium.[20] The presence of levonorgestrel causes a high expression of insulin-like growth factor (IGF) binding protein-1 in the endometrium, which inhibits the activity of IGF-1. IGF-1 is thought to mediate the mitogenic action of estrogens. Inhibition of its activity causes suppression of endometrial proliferation.[25]

EFFECT ON CERVICAL MUCUS

The intrauterine release of levonorgestrel is also found to affect cervical mucus. It is a common clinical observation that cervical mucus is very scarce and viscous in LNG-IUS users. Analysis of the properties of the mucus during intrauterine levonorgestrel administration shows that the water content in relation to mucin concentration is much lower than during use of copper-releasing IUDs.[10] This phenomenon is thought at least partly to inhibit sperm migration through the cervical canal and thus contribute to the contraceptive effect of the LNG-IUS.

EFFECT ON OVARIAN FUNCTION

It is possible to cause suppression of ovulation by intrauterine administration of levonorgestrel.

However, suppression of ovulation is not the mechanism by which the high contraceptive effectiveness of Mirena®, the LNG-IUS releasing 20µg per 24h, is achieved. In fact, the incidence of anovulatory cycles in Mirena® users does not differ from that registered during use of copper-releasing IUDs.[5,28] In dose-finding studies during the early development of the LNG-IUS, it was shown that intrauterine release rates associated with plasma concentrations of levonorgestrel less than 200pg ml^{-1} did not affect ovulation.[16] Mirena® releases 20µg per day of levonorgestrel, which corresponds to an average plasma concentration of 150pg ml^{-1}. The low circulating concentrations of levonorgestrel have, however, some effects on ovarian function that might contribute to the contraceptive effectiveness.

Overall, progesterone concentrations during the luteal phase of the cycle are lower in Mirena® users than in users of inert or copper-releasing IUDs.[5,7] On the other hand, estradiol concentrations during the menstrual cycle are not affected by the use of Mirena®.[7]

Demonstrating chorionic activity by the presence of human chorionic gonadotropin (hCG) in the blood circulation of users of inert and copper-releasing IUDs suggests that these IUDs do not necessarily prevent fertilisation and that their mechanism of action might even include an abortifacient component.[15,33] Detectable concentrations of hCG have not been found during use of LNG-IUS.[33] Examinations of ova recovered from the fallopian tubes of humans using different kinds of intrauterine contraception showed no development of the ova during use of the LNG-IUS.[23] These findings suggest that LNG-IUS prevents fertilisation.

CONTRACEPTIVE EFFECTIVENESS OF MIRENA®

In order to get an accurate picture of the contraceptive effectiveness and the acceptability of use of a new contraceptive method comparative studies should be undertaken, using well-established and effective methods as a reference point. Reports on several randomised comparative studies with Mirena® compared with copper-releasing IUDs, such as the Nova-T®, the CuT 380Ag, the CuT 200 and the CuT 220, have been published. A common feature of these studies is a significantly lower rate of accidental pregnancies in Mirena® users. Table 4.1 summarises the pregnancy rates of these reports.

The first randomised study compared LNG-IUSs releasing 20 and 30µg with the Nova-T® copper-releasing IUD. This blinded trial recruited 321 women who were followed for three years.[17]

Table 4.1 Gross cumulative pregnancy rates in four randomised clinical trials comparing the levonorgestrel-releasing intrauterine system (LNG-IUS) with different copper-releasing IUDs (Cu-IUD)

Trial		Number of women	Follow-up (years)	Pregnancy rate
Nilsson et al[17]	LNG-IUS	321	2	0.6
	Cu-IUD	321	2	3.3
Andersson et al[4]	LNG-IUS	1821	5	0.5
	Cu-IUD	937	5	5.9
Sivin et al[30]	LNG-IUS	1124	5	1.1
	Cu-IUD	1121	5	1.4
Indian CMR[9]	LNG-IUS	475	3	0.0
	Cu-IUD	500	3	1.6

After two years it was clear that the system releasing 30 μg per day offered no advantage over the one releasing 20 μg per day. The pregnancy and expulsion rates were significantly lower with Mirena® users than in the Nova-T® users.[21] The most important study is a European multicentre study, involving a total of 2758 women in 14 centres in Denmark, Finland, Hungary, Norway and Sweden. The randomisation between Mirena® and Nova-T® was 2 : 1 in favour of Mirena® and the study lasted for five years. The differences in pregnancy rates between the two devices were highly significant; at one year $p < 0.006$ and at three and five years $p < 0.001$. The pregnancy rates in different age groups among the Nova-T® users followed the expected pattern of showing the highest rate of 14.9 in the youngest age group (< 25 years) with declining rates of 6.9 (26–30 years), 4.0 (31–35 years) and 2.8 in the older age groups (> 35 years), respectively. The age-dependant fertility effect was completely abolished in Mirena® users with no pregnancies in the youngest age group and the highest rate of 0.9 in the oldest age group. In a multicentre study in India, involving 1905 women, Mirena® was compared with three different copper-releasing IUDs: the CuT 200, CuT 220 and CuT 380Ag. The observation period was three years during which time no pregnancies were observed with Mirena® during 10 500 women-months of use, while the pregnancy rates varied between 0.3 and 1.6 with the copper-releasing devices.[9] In yet another randomised multicentre study Mirena® was compared to the CuT 389Ag device.

Of the initial 2244 women, 1793 women elected to continue in the study for seven years. The seven-year gross cumulative pregnancy rates per 100 women users were 1.1 for Mirena® and 1.4 for CuT 380Ag.[30]

ECTOPIC PREGNANCIES

The risk of ectopic pregnancies has been a cause of concern with the IUDs in the past. The risk of ectopic pregnancy is related to the contraceptive effectiveness of the device. IUDs prevent intrauterine pregnancies more effectively than they prevent ectopic pregnancies. The rate of ectopic pregnancies during IUD use is, however, lower than observed in an unprotected population.

The progesterone-releasing Progestasert® was withdrawn from the market because of the unacceptably high rate of ectopic pregnancies that was reported in association with its use.

In the large European multicentre study, the cumulative rate of ectopic pregnancies after five years of follow-up was 0.02 per 100 women months of use for Mirena® and 0.25 for the Nova-T®, the difference being statistically significant. Compared with the rates of ectopic pregnancies of 1.2–1.6 occurring in sexually active unprotected women, the rates associated with Mirena® have to be regarded as extremely low and the fact acknowledged that Mirena® offers protection against ectopic pregnancies.

Altogether Mirena® has been associated with significantly lower pregnancy rates in randomised clinical trials than any other IUD with which it has been compared. It is the most effective reversible contraceptive method, even more effective, in fact, than female tubal ligation.

BLEEDING CONTROL DURING MIRENA® USE

DURING CONTRACEPTIVE USE

Intermenstrual spotting is a common feature with progestin-only contraceptive methods. Irregular bleeding and intermenstrual spotting were reported to occur in 20–30% of women using Progestasert®. In the first randomised comparative trial comparing Mirena® to Nova-T® it was found that the total number of days of menstrual bleeding was significantly lower in Mirena® users than in Nova-T® users from the time of insertion of the IUDs to the end of the first year of treatment. The number of days of intermenstrual spotting was higher during the first three months of treatment in Mirena® users than in Nova-T® users, but thereafter significantly lower in Mirena® users. During the five years of follow-up in the European multicentre study the termination rates due to bleeding problems were equal for both Mirena® and Nova-T® during the first year of treatment. Thereafter the termination rates due to bleeding problems were increasingly higher in the Nova-T® group towards the end of five years of treatment. The cumulative five-year gross rates of termination due to bleeding problems were significantly lower in the Mirena® group compared with the Nova-T® group, 13.7 and 20.9 respectively. Figure 4.1 shows the mean number of days of bleeding and spotting during the first year of use of the two devices.

A reduction in the amount of blood loss during treatment with intrauterine levonorgestrel was observed at an early stage of development of the levonorgestrel-releasing intrauterine system. A comparative quantitation of the total amount of blood loss, including both menstrual bleeding and intermenstrual spotting, showed that already after the first month of treatment a significant decrease in blood loss could be measured in the LNG-IUS users while a significant increase in blood loss was seen in the Nova-T® users. The haemoglobin concentration of peripheral blood increased significantly during three months' treatment with the LNG-IUS.[14]

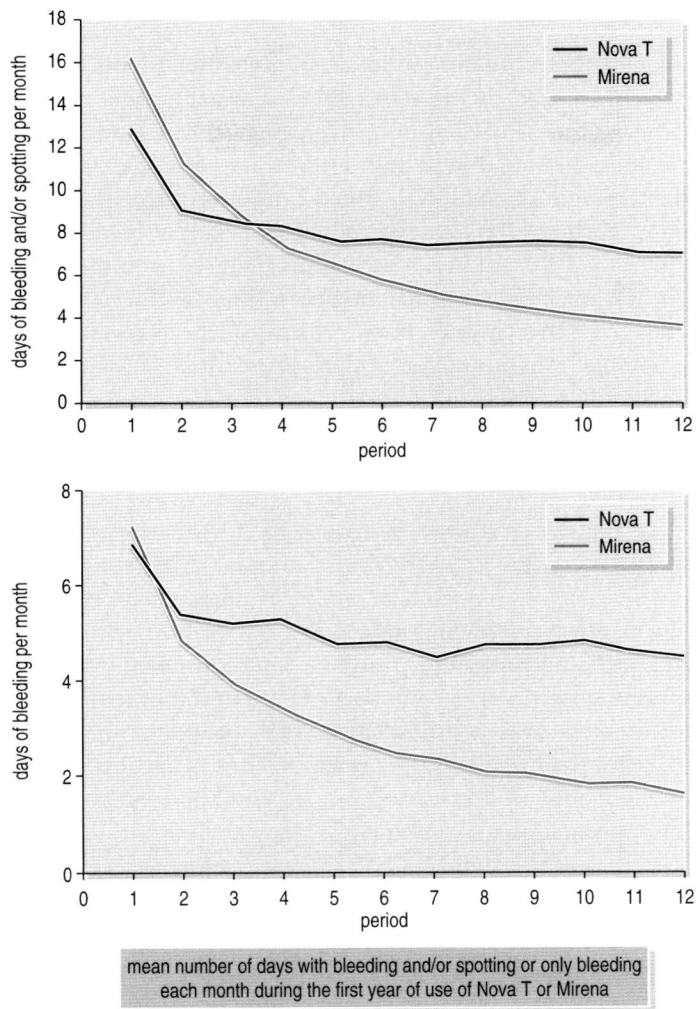

Fig 4.1 European Multicentre Study: patterns of bleeding.
Mean number of days with bleeding and/or spotting or only bleeding each month during the first year of use of Nova-T® or Mirena®.
(© 1994 Mirena Training Programme, Pharmacia-Leiras BV)

The local effect on the endometrium by the released levonorgestrel is the cause of the reduced blood loss. A certain proportion of Mirena® users develops a state of local amenorrhoea. Depending on how amenorrhoea is defined, between 20 and 30% of the users develop amenorrhoea during the first year of treatment. An additional 10 to 15% experienced amenorrhoea later on during treatment. The state of amenorrhoea is not a reflection of ovarian function. There is no difference in ovulatory behaviour between women menstruating or developing amenorrhoea during Mirena® use.[22]

DURING TREATMENT OF MENORRHAGIA

The observation of the profound reduction in menstrual blood loss during use of Mirena® has been utilised in the effort to treat menorrhagia. In a series of 20 women with heavy menstrual bleeding, averaging 200 ml, Andersson et al measured an 86% reduction in blood loss after three months of treatment with Mirena® and a final reduction of 97% after 12 months of treatment.[1] In the study by Andersson et al the blood loss was reduced to normal levels even in women with menstrual blood loss as heavy as 400 ml. The reduced blood loss was followed by a significant increase in haemoglobin levels and in serum ferritin concentrations. Several other studies have confirmed these results. In a study by Milsom et al, Mirena® was compared to flurbiprofen (an NSAID) and tranexamic acid (an antifibrinolytic drug) in the treatment of menorrhagia. They found that blood loss was reduced by 20% with flurbiprofen treatment and 40% with tranexamic acid treatment while blood loss was reduced by 80–90% with the use of Mirena®.[12]

RETURN OF FERTILITY

The strong local effect of levonorgestrel on the endometrium during use of Mirena® could potentially affect or postpone the return of fertility after removal of the intrauterine system. At an early stage of the development of the LNG-IUS return of fertility was registered in a small series of women having their LNG-IUS removed because of planned pregnancy. Return of fertility was found to be normal and conception even occurred in a few of the women during the first cycle after discontinuation of treatment.[19] Two review articles conclude that pregnancy rates after removal of Mirena® are comparable to those in women who have not used any form of contraception.[6,32]

In a larger study, which was part of the European multicentre study, users of both Mirena® and Nova-T® who had their devices removed for planned pregnancy were followed after discontinuation. Not only pregnancy but also the outcomes of the first pregnancy were evaluated. The women were followed for at least 24 months or to term. There were no statistical differences in age, parity, obstetrical history, incidence of PID or duration of IUD use between the 138 former Mirena® users and the 71 Nova-T® users. During the follow-up period 75.4% of the former Mirena® users and 70.4% of the former Nova-T® users became pregnant. Among those who conceived, 92% in both groups became pregnant during the first year after device removal. There was no significant difference in the pregnancy rate between the two devices. Duration of use before removal did not affect the conception rate.[2] There was no difference in the outcome of pregnancy between the groups, the rate of live births being equal. There were no stillbirths in the Mirena® group and only two in the Nova-T® group. After removal of Mirena® for planned pregnancy, conception occurred within the same time period as after removal of any other intrauterine device or as in women who have not used any kind of protection.

HORMONAL EFFECTS OF INTRAUTERINE LEVONORGESTREL RELEASE

Mirena® releasing 20 μg levonorgestrel per day is a hormonal method of preventing pregnancy. The hormonal effect is mainly local on the endometrium. Only a small proportion of the levonorgestrel released in utero can be detected in peripheral blood, the average concentration being around 150 pg ml^{-1}. These plasma levels are only a quarter of the mean levels of the lowest oral progestin-only pills. The main hormonal side effects registered mostly during the first three months after insertion of Mirena® are: acne, nausea, headache, depression and breast tenderness.

In the European multicentre study no difference in measured weight gain was found between Mirena® and Nova-T® users. Significant differences in cumulative gross termination rates for hormonal reasons, such as depression, acne, headache and weight gain, were reported in the multicentre study. In one study, women were asked 12 months after the insertion of either a Mirena® or a Nova-T® device to compare the present method with their previous IUD. More than 70% of Mirena® users were more satisfied with Mirena® than with their previous IUD, and less than 5% were less satisfied.[27]

Levonorgestrel is a 19-nortestosteron derivative and has certain androgenic effects on lipid metabolism. During contraceptive use of Mirena® no differences in total cholesterol, HDL-cholesterol or triglycerides were registered compared with women using a copper-releasing IUD in a cross-sectional study.[18] In a longitudinal study of perimenopausal women on estrogen substitution with a Mirena® inserted for the purpose of endometrial protection no changes in total cholesterol, HDL-cholesterol, LDL-cholesterol or triglycerides compared with baseline values were found after 12 months of treatment.[3]

In the 1970s, at the time when the development of the LNG-IUS was initiated it was believed that the use of intrauterine devices for contraceptive purposes increased the risk of pelvic inflammatory disease (PID). On the other hand there were reports suggesting that the use of the oral combined contraceptive pill was associated with a slight protective effect against PID. In the five-year European multicentre study a significantly lower rate of PID in the Mirena® group compared with the Nova-T® group was seen at three years of follow-up and this finding was further confirmed at the five-year follow-up. An interesting and reassuring feature of this protective effect of Mirena® was that the greatest difference in PID rate was seen in the youngest age group, which is usually at the highest risk of acquiring PID.

HEALTH BENEFITS

PREGNANCY ASSOCIATED

Through its high effectiveness in preventing pregnancy, Mirena® averts pregnancy-associated morbidity, such as sepsis in association with illegal abortions, first and second trimester mortality and mortality associated with delivery especially in developing countries. During the use of Mirena® there is a 90%

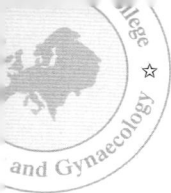

reduction in the expected rate of ectopic pregnancies compared with women who employ no method of contraception and the rate is markedly lower than ectopic pregnancy rates associated with the use of barrier methods.[8] The possibility of adequately treating cases of ectopic pregnancy in developing countries is poor and thus any method of contraception that substantially decreases the risk of ectopic pregnancies will have a marked effect on the health of fertile women.

BLEEDING ASSOCIATED

As Mirena® already very profoundly reduces both the volume and the duration of menstrual bleeding within 2–6 months following insertion the effect on haemoglobin levels and serum ferritin concentrations during long-term use has a significant impact on women's health in both developed and especially developing countries. In cases of anaemia due to menorrhagia the more than 90% reduction in blood loss during treatment with Mirena® offers a significant improvement over several alternative treatment modalities. In a Finnish open randomised study, 56 women who were scheduled for hysterectomy because of menorrhagia either continued with their current medical treatment or had a Mirena® inserted. After six months 67% of the women in the Mirena® group cancelled their operation compared with 14% in the control group.

There was a significant rise in the haemoglobin concentration of the Mirena® group and a significant improvement in quality of life compared with the situation before insertion and compared with the control group.[11] Thus Mirena® seems to be an effective, very acceptable and non-invasive way of treating menorrhagia in cases where hysterectomy has been suggested.

IN ASSOCIATION WITH DYSMENORRHOEA

In a study comparing Mirena® with a copper-releasing IUD it was found that pre-insertion menstrual pain was reduced significantly during a one-year treatment period in the Mirena® group while no changes in the experience of dysmenorrhoea were found in the copper-releasing IUD group. In the same study symptoms of premenstrual discomfort were registered. There was a significant decrease of premenstrual symptoms in the Mirena® group with no change of symptoms in the copper-releasing IUD group.[28]

IN ASSOCIATION WITH HORMONE REPLACEMENT THERAPY

Unopposed estrogen replacement therapy is associated with the risk of endometrial hyperplasia, adenomatous changes and even endometrial carcinoma. Traditionally, the addition of monthly oral progestin treatment for ten days has been thought to effectively avoid this risk. However, cyclic oral progestin treatment causes regular menstrual-like bleeding in postmenopausal women, which often interferes with compliance. The estrogenic effect on the endometrium is opposed by the local release of levonorgestrel much more effectively than by any other route of administration because of the high concentrations achieved in the endometrium. This finding has been utilised in the treatment of established endometrial hyperplasia.[26] The rapid remission of hyperplasia indicates that the progestin concentration in the endometrium is correlated with the degree of endometrial protection. Mirena® has been approved on the market as a method of protecting the endometrium during postmenopausal estrogen replacement therapy.

In a prospective, multicentre, seven-year randomised study Mirena® was compared with the CuT 380Ag device for adverse events. During 3416 women years of Mirena® use only one case of uterine myoma was found while 14 cases were detected in the copper IUD group during 3975 years of use. This difference is significant and the incidence of myomas in the copper IUD group increased with time and resulted in surgical treatment in six of the cases while no surgery was needed in the Mirena® group.[31] It thus seems as if the use of a levonorgestrel-releasing intrauterine system has the ability to decrease the risk of developing uterine myomas.

SUMMARY

The levonorgestrel-releasing intrauterine system has become the most important method for intrauterine medication. Mirena® can be successfully used throughout the reproductive period for effective contraception. Furthermore, women fitted with the system experience additional health benefits in terms of favourable effects on dysmenorrhoea, premenstrual symptoms, menstrual blood loss, lower risk of PID and incidence of uterine myomas. Mirena® has proved to be the most effective medical treatment of idiopathic menorrhagia and is an alternative to hysterectomy in cases of heavy bleeding problems.

References

1. Andersson K, Rybo G 1990 Levonorgestrel intrauterine device in the treatment of menorrhagia. British Journal of Obstetrics and Gynaecology 97:690–694

2. Andersson K, Batar I, Rybo G 1992 Return of fertility after removal of a levonorgestrel-releasing device and Nova-T. Contraception 46:575–584

3. Andersson K, Stadberg E, Mattson L-Å, Rybo G, Samsioe G 1996 Intrauterine or oral administration of levonorgestrel in combination with estradiol for climacteric complaints: effect on lipid metabolism during 12 months of treatment. International Journal of Fertility and Menopausal Studies 41:476–483

4. Andersson K, Odlind V, Rybo G 1994 Levonorgestrel-releasing and copper-releasing (Nova-T) IUDs during five years of use. Contraception 49:56–72

5. Barbosa I, Bakos O, Olsson S-E, Odlind V, Johansson E D B 1990 Ovarian function during use of a levonorgestrel-releasing IUD. Contraception 42:51–66.

6. Coleman M, McCovan L, Farquhar C 1997 The levonorgestrel-releasing intrauterine device: a wider role than contraception. Australian and New Zealand Journal of Obstetrics and Gynecology 37:195–201

7. Doyle L L, Clewe T H 1968 Preliminary studies on the effect of hormone-releasing intrauterine devices. American Journal of Obstetrics and Gynecology 101:564–568

8. Gray R H 1985 A case-controlled study of ectopic pregnancy in developed and developing countries In: Zatuchni G, Goldsmith A, Sciarra J J (eds) Intrauterine contraception: advances and future concepts. Harper & Row, Philadelphia, pp 354–364

9. Indian Council of Medical Research Task Force on IUD 1989 Randomised clinical

trial with intrauterine devices (levonorgestrel intrauterine device (LNG), CuT 380Ag, CuT 220C and CuT 200B). A 36-month study. Contraception 39:37–52

10. Jonsson B, Landgren B M, Eneroth P 1991 Effects of various IUDs on the composition of cervical mucus. Contraception 43:447–458

11. Lähteenmäki P, Haukkamaa M, Puolakka J, Riikonen U, Sainio S, Suvisaari J, Nilsson C G 1998 Open randomised study of use of levonorgestrel-releasing intrauterine system as an alternative to hysterectomy. British Medical Journal 316:1122–1126

12. Milsom I, Andersson K, Andersch B, Rybo G 1991 A comparison of flurbiprofen, tranexamic acid and a levonorgestrel-releasing intrauterine device in the treatment of idiopathic menorrhagia. American Journal of Obstetrics and Gynecology 164:879–883

13. Nilsson C G, Luukkainen T, Lähteenmäki P 1977 Contraception with a norethisterone-releasing IUD: plasma levels of norethisterone and its influence on the ovarian function. Contraception 17:115–122

14. Nilsson C G 1977 Comparative quantitation of menstrual blood loss with a d-norgestrel-releasing IUD and a Nova-T copper device. Contraception 15:379–387

15. Nilsson C G, Lähteenmäki P, Luukkainen T 1979 Detection of beta subunit hCG in plasma of IUD users as an indication of frequency of conception. International Journal of Fertility 24:134–137

16. Nilsson C G, Lähteenmäki P, Robertson D N, Luukkainen T 1980 Plasma concentrations of levonorgestrel as a function of the release rate of levonorgestrel from a medicated intrauterine device. Acta Endocrinol 93:380–384

17. Nilsson C G, Luukkainen T, Diaz J, Allonen H 1981 Intrauterine contraception with levonorgestrel: a comparative randomised clinical performance study. Lancet i:577–580

18. Nilsson C G, Kostiainen E, Ehnholm C 1981 Serum lipids and high-density lipoprotein-cholesterol in women on long-term sustained low-dose IUD treatment with levonorgestrel. International Journal of Fertility 26:135–137

19. Nilsson C G 1982 Fertility after discontinuation of levonorgestrel-releasing intrauterine devices. Contraception 25:273–278

20. Nilsson C G, Haukkamaa M, Vierola H, Luukkainen T 1982 Tissue concentrations of levonorgestrel in women using a levonorgestrel-releasing IUD. Clinical Endocrinology 17:529–536

21. Nilsson C G, Allonen H, Diaz J, Luukkainen T 1983 Two years' experience with two levonorgestrel-releasing intrauterine devices and one copper-releasing intrauterine device. A randomised comparative performance study. Fertility and Sterility 39:187–192

22. Nilsson C G, Löhteenmäki P L A, Luukkainen T 1984 Ovarian function in amenorrheic and menstruating users of a levonorgestrel-releasing intrauterine device. Fertility and Sterility 41:52–55

23. Ortiz M E, Croxatto H B 1987 The mode of action of IUDs. Contraception 36:37–53

24. Rudel H W, Martinez-Manautou J, Maqueo-Topete M 1965 The role of progestogens in the hormonal control of fertility. Fertility and Sterility 16:158–167

25. Rutanen E M, Salmi A, Nyman T 1997 mRNA expression of insulin-like growth factor-I (IGF-I) is suppressed and those of IGF-II and IGF-binding protein-I are constantly expressed in the endometrium during use of an intrauterine levonorgestrel system. Molecular Human Reproduction 3:749–754

26. Scarselli G, Tantini C, Colafranceschi M 1988 Levonorgestrel-Nova-T and precancerous lesions of the endometrium. European Journal of Gynecological Oncology 9:284–286

27. Schain R N, Ratsula K, Toivonen J, Lähteenmäki P, Luukkainen T, Holden A E C, Rosenthal M 1989 Acceptability of an experimental intracervical device: results of a study controlling for selection bias. Contraception 39:73–84

28. Scholten P C, Christiaens G C M L, Haspels A A 1989 Treatment of menorrhagia by intrauterine administration of levonorgestrel. In: Scholten P C The Levonorgestrel IUD. Thesis, Utrecht University Hospital, Utrecht

29. Sivergerg S G, Haukkamaa M, Arko H, Nilsson C G, Luukkainen T 1986 Endometrial morphology during long-term use of levonorgestrel-releasing intrauterine devices. International Journal of Gynecological Pathology 5:235–241

30. Sivin I, Stern J, Coutinho E et al 1991 Prolonged intrauterine contraception: a seven-year randomized study of the levonorgestrel 20 mcg/day (LNg 20) and Copper T380Ag IUDS. Contraception 44:473–480

31. Sivin I, Stern J 1994 Health during prolonged use of levonorgestrel 20 mcg/day and copper CuT 380Ag intrauterine contraceptive devices: a multicenter study. Fertility and Sterility 61:70–77

32. Sturridge F, Guillebaud J 1996 A risk-benefit assessment of the levonorgestrel-releasing intrauterine system. Drug Safety 15:430–440

33. Videla-Rivero L, Etchepareborda J J, Kesserü E 1987 Early chorionic activity in women bearing inert IUD, copper IUD and levonorgestrel-releasing IUD. Contraception 36:217–226

34. World Health Organization, Special Programme of Research Development and Research Training in Human Reproduction 1983 The Alza T IPCS 52, a longer acting progesterone IUD: safety and efficacy compared to the CuT220C and Multiload 250 in two randomized multicentre trials. Clinical Reproduction and Fertility 2:113–128

5

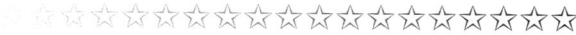
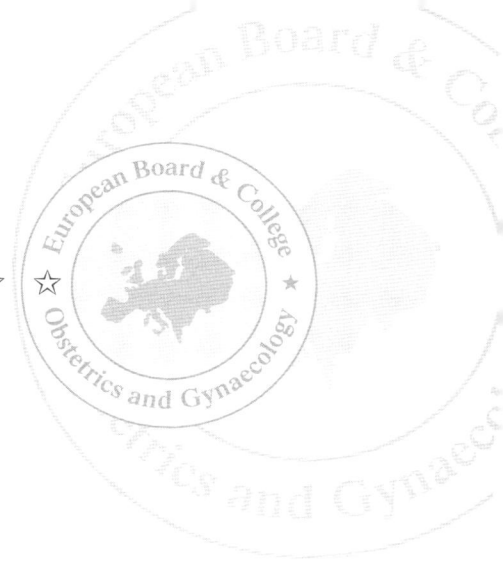

Spermicidal and barrier methods of contraception

Mary Short

ABSTRACT

Barrier contraception provides a mechanical barrier to prevent transportation of sperm, thus preventing fertilisation. Barrier and spermicidal methods have been in circulation since ancient times with everything from lemon juice to camel dung being used to prevent sperm penetration. Examples of barrier contraceptives include the male condom, the female condom, and the diaphragm. To date barrier devices are the only contraceptive methods that can help prevent the spread of STDs.

KEYWORDS

Barrier contraception, spermicide, male and female condom, diaphragm, cervical cap, microbicides.

SPERMICIDES

Spermicides[6,21,28] are sperm-killing substances available as foams, creams, or gels, and are often used in female contraception with barrier and other devices. Spermicides are usually available without prescription or medical examination.

The active ingredient in US-made spermicides is usually nonoxynol-9, which attacks the surface of the sperm cell. Nonoxynol-9, however, does not provide any additional protection against sexually transmitted diseases.[18] In fact, research now suggests that frequent use may cause vaginal injuries and actually increase the risk for HIV transmission in women. In addition, use of a spermicide with a barrier device also poses a two- to three-fold risk for a urinary tract infection in women, regardless of whether the device is a condom or diaphragm. Spermicides are no longer recommended with male condoms. Some experts question their use with the diaphragm, suggesting that they may not even add much protection against pregnancies.[35] A major analysis of current research found only one study that reported enhanced protection, but it had limitations.[14]

In general, spermicides may be an appropriate choice for women who have intercourse only once in a while, or need backup protection against pregnancy (for instance, if they forget to take their birth-control pills). Spermicides should not be used alone as the primary method of birth control. Nor should they be used to prevent sexually transmitted diseases.

DIAPHRAGM

The diaphragm, which is generally used with a spermicidal cream, foam, or gel, is a small convex-shaped latex device with a flexible ring that fits over the cervix and is held in place by its rim, which fits snugly under the pubic symphysis. It acts as a physical barrier against the transport of sperm into the uterus. The use of spermicides with a diaphragm is under debate. They may not offer additional protection against pregnancy, can increase the risk of urinary tract infections, and do not protect against sexually transmitted diseases. Although traditionally the spermicide is considered to provide additional chemical protection.

The diaphragm is self inserted over the cervix prior to intercourse and is left in place several hours after intercourse.

There are three basic rim designs.

- The Arcing Spring diaphragm applies strong pressure and easily flips into place. It is useful for women with weak vaginal muscles and for new users who are worried about incorrect placement.
- The Coil Spring Rim is useful for women with strong vaginal muscles.
- The Flat Spring Rim has a delicate rim and a gentle spring, and may be appropriate for women who have not had children.

Diaphragms come in different sizes from 60 mm, increasing in diameter at 5 mm intervals, and require a fitting by a trained health-care provider who prescribes the correct size of diaphragm for the user and instructs her in the use of the diaphragm. Some women will need to be refitted with a different-sized diaphragm after pregnancy, abdominal or pelvic surgery, or weight loss or gain of 4.5 kg or more. As a general rule, diaphragms should be replaced every one to two years.

Although the diaphragm has a relatively high failure rate, even with perfect use, it is considered a good choice for women whose health or lifestyle prevents them from using more effective hormonal contraceptives. Certain conditions of the vagina and uterus, or a history of recurrent urinary tract infections, may disqualify a woman from using the device. The diaphragm should not be used if either partner is allergic to latex or spermicides.

USING AND INSERTING THE DIAPHRAGM

The diaphragm may be placed in the vagina any time before intercourse and can be used even when a woman is menstruating.[16,24] However if the diaphragm is in situ for more than six hours additional spermicide should be employed.

General guidelines for insertion:

1. Before or after each use, the woman should hold the diaphragm up to the light or fill it with water to check for holes, tears or leaks.
2. A small amount of spermicide (about one teaspoon) is usually placed inside the diaphragm, and some is smeared around its rim.
3. The device is then folded in half and inserted into the vagina by hand or with assistance of a plastic inserter.
4. The diaphragm should fit over the cervix, blocking entry to the cervix (neck of womb).
5. If more than six hours pass before repeat intercourse occurs, the diaphragm is left in place and extra spermicide is inserted into the vagina using an applicator.
6. The diaphragm must remain in the vagina for six to eight hours after the final act of intercourse, and can safely stay there up to 24 hours after insertion.
7. The diaphragm should be washed with soap and warm water after each use and then stored in its original container, which should be kept in a cool dry place.

ADVANTAGES OF THE DIAPHRAGM

The diaphragm is easily portable and can be inserted at a convenient time before intercourse begins. It is therefore independent of coital activity. Generally speaking it cannot be felt by either partner. It appears to protect against cervical gonorrhoea, chlamydia and trichomoniasis, although more research is needed to confirm this. It does not provide protection against sexually transmitted infections in areas other than the cervix.

DISADVANTAGES OF THE DIAPHRAGM

1. Failure rates vary greatly; figures of 5–20% have been quoted.
2. Some women dislike having to insert the device every time intercourse occurs or have trouble mastering the insertion and removal process.
3. Recurrent urinary tract infections may pose a problem for some. Resizing and voiding before and after coital activity reduces the incidence of UTIs.
4. Rare cases of toxic shock syndrome have been reported among diaphragm users. To be safe, the diaphragm should not stay in place for more than 24 hours.
5. It is still important for effective contraception to retain the diaphragm for six to eight hours after intercourse.

CERVICAL CAP

The cervical cap (Prentif®, FemCap®) is a thimble or dome-shaped latex cup that fits over the cervix and is always used with a spermicidal cream or gel.[7,9,37,39] It is held in place by the suction created between the cervix and the cap. It is like the diaphragm but smaller, and is available in only four sizes. The cap is available by prescription and requires a pelvic examination and sizing, as well as instruction by a health-care provider.

INSERTION AND USE OF THE CERVICAL CAP

A small amount of spermicide is placed in the cap, the device is then inserted manually. As in diaphragm use, instruction and practice is required. The cap must be kept in the vagina for eight hours after intercourse. Caps should be replaced every one to two years. A refitting may be needed after pregnancy or cervical surgery.

SUITABILITY OF THE CERVICAL CAP

Because of the restricted range of available sizes, about one woman in five will not be suitable to be fitted for the cap.

1. Abnormal cervical cytology.
2. A history of toxic shock syndrome.
3. A current sexually transmitted or reproductive tract infection.
4. Untreated cervicitis.

ADVANTAGES OF THE CERVICAL CAP

1. No association with UTI.
2. No association with toxic shock syndrome.
3. May be left in situ 48 hours after intercourse.
4. No additional spermicide required.

DISADVANTAGES OF THE CERVICAL CAP

1. Failure rate is high (higher than all other methods of contraception). In general, the FemCap® has a higher risk for failure than either the diaphragm or the Prentif® cap.
2. Unlike the diaphragm, the cap cannot be used during menstruation, although there are no associated problems with the start of menstruation while the cap is in situ.

FEMALE CONDOM

The female condom (e.g. Reality®, Femidom®) is a lubricated, polyurethane, loose-fitting pouch containing two flexible rings to hold it in place.[17,25,32,33,46] It is designed to line the vagina and create a physical barrier against sperm and sexually transmitted diseases by surrounding the penis and the external female genitalia during intercourse. It should be used independently of other methods of contraception, particularly a male condom.

The failure rate for the female condom is about the same as for the diaphragm and cervical cap. It is available without a prescription.[3,5]

USE AND INSERTION OF THE FEMALE CONDOM

The female condom is about 7.5 cm wide and approximately 15 cm long (larger than a male condom), with a flexible ring at both ends.[15,19]

1. The ring at the closed end is used to insert the device into the vagina and hold it in place over the cervix. (However, this ring may be removed if the woman finds it too uncomfortable.)
2. The ring at the open end remains outside the vagina and partly covers the labia.
3. The female condom is inserted manually into the vagina up to eight hours before intercourse.
4. Although the female condom is prelubricated, extra lubricant is sometimes needed while inserting the device or during intercourse.
5. As the female condom is made from polyurethane, oil-based lubricants may be used.
6. The woman checks to be sure that the outer ring is lying flat against her labia guiding her partner's penis into the ring.

The female condom should be removed and a new one inserted if there are any tears, the outer ring descends into the vagina or any bunching of the condom occurs in the vagina.[40,41,42,43]

The female condom may be the contraceptive of choice for women who are not certain that their male partner will use a condom. There are no contraindications to its usage although uptake is poor due to aesthetic perceptions.

ADVANTAGES OF THE FEMALE CONDOM

1. The female condom affords some protection against sexually transmitted diseases, since it covers a large area, including external genitalia. However, there are few clinical studies at this time to determine this protection against sexually transmitted diseases.[10]
2. The standard female condom is made of polyurethane, which is thin and soft but at the same time 40% stronger than the latex male condoms.
3. Polyurethane is not damaged by lubricating oils, and is less likely to cause an allergic reaction.
4. It transmits body heat better than latex, softening the condom and providing a more natural sensation.
5. Immediate penile withdrawal is not essential.

DISADVANTAGES AND COMPLICATIONS OF THE FEMALE CONDOM

1. Compliance rates are low for many reasons.[29]
2. About 25% of women have difficulty on the first attempt at self-insertion.
3. Some women find the condom aesthetically displeasing and therefore they are not suitable candidates for female condom usage. The inner ring may be uncomfortable for some women (in which case it can be removed).

4. It may be noisy at the commencement of intercourse and without sufficient lubrication, it can also be pushed out of place by the penis. Using more lubricant can help keep the female condom in place and reduce the noise.

THE MALE CONDOM

The condom is still the only reversible form of male contraception currently available.[23,34]

PREGNANCY PROTECTION

The condom should be put on before intercourse when the penis is erect, since sufficient semen may be leaked before ejaculation occurs to result in pregnancy. The average rate of pregnancy for couples that rely only on condoms for protection is higher (about 12%). In adolescents the risk with condoms is even higher (18%). Even for those who use a good-quality condom correctly, the annual risk for pregnancy is 3%.

PREVENTION OF SEXUALLY TRANSMITTED DISEASES

Condoms are important in the reduction of transmission of sexually transmitted diseases in both male and female partners but they have limitations.[1,2,4,27,30,44,45] In men they are more protective against seminal-fluid-transmitted infections (e.g. gonorrhoea, chlamydia, trichomoniasis and HIV) than in preventing those transmitted by skin-to-skin contact (e.g. herpes simplex virus, HPV, syphilis and chancroid). Male condoms, in fact, offer better protection against herpes for women than they do for men. (Men often shed the virus from the skin of the penis, which is covered by the condom. In women the virus is often shed from areas around the genitals, which can contact male skin outside the condom.)

Some condoms come prelubricated with spermicide nonoxynol-9, which is no longer recommended with condoms because of a lack of protection and a higher risk for HIV infection. Its use in male condoms also promotes yeast and urinary tract infections in women.

A unique synthetic polymer gel (PRO 2000 Gel) interferes with viral infection itself—not the sperm—and is undergoing trials. Early studies suggest that it is well tolerated, although it does have some adverse effects, including vaginal discharge and bleeding.

CONDOM MATERIALS

1. *Latex*. Condoms made of latex rubber are the most common types.[38] They are less likely to slip or break than those made of polyurethane (Avanti® or eZ-on®), and they are contoured for better fit thus providing fairly effective protection. Some people are allergic to latex. The latex smell may also be unpleasant for some people.[12,13]

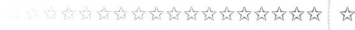

2. *Polyurethane*. Polyurethane condoms (Avanti®, eZ-on®) are now available. It is hoped that eventually they will prove to be superior to latex in a number of ways, including strength, sensitivity, and durability. At this point, they have had good acceptance by couples but have a higher breakage rate (6–7.2%) compared with the latex condom (1.1–2%). Other synthetic materials are under investigation.
3. *Animal membranes*. Condoms made from animal membrane can prevent pregnancy, but sexually transmitted infections can permeate them.

THE SPONGE

The sponge (Protectaid®, Today®) is a disposable form of barrier contraception.[20] It is made of soft polyurethane, is round in shape, and it fits over the cervix like a diaphragm, but it is smaller and easily portable. The Today® sponge contains ten-times the amount of the spermicide, nonoxynol-9, than other products. The Protectaid® sponge is currently available in Canada; it contains a mix of three spermicides (nonoxynol-9, sodium cholate and benzalkonium chloride).

USE AND INSERTION

To use the sponge, the woman first wets it with water, then inserts it into the vagina with a finger, using a cord loop attachment. It can be inserted up to six hours before intercourse and should be left in place for at least six hours following intercourse. The sponge provides protection for up to 12 hours. It should not be left in for more than 30 hours from time of insertion.

The sponge should not be used during menstruation, after childbirth, or by women with a history of toxic shock syndrome.

ADVANTAGES OF THE SPONGE

Because the sponge is not felt during intercourse, it encourages spontaneity. It appears to protect against cervical gonorrhoea and chlamydia.

DISADVANTAGES OF THE SPONGE

Failure rates (about 10%) are higher than with the diaphragm. There is a very small risk for toxic shock using the sponge, as there is for other barrier methods of contraception. People who are allergic to spermicides should not use the sponge. The sponge does not protect against HIV or sexually transmitted diseases outside the cervix. It increases the risk for candidiasis (yeast infection).

LEA SHIELD

The Lea shield is made of silicone and its cup-shaped bowl completely surrounds the cervix without resting on it.[26,31] The shield, therefore, does not need to be fitted, and manufacturers showed results equal to the diaphragm and cap when used with spermicide.

Its advantages are as follows:

1. One size fits all.
2. Can be left for up to 48 hours after intercourse.
3. Reusable for six months.

MICROBICIDES

With almost 34 million people worldwide living with HIV/AIDS—95% of whom are in developing countries—the need for additional prevention options has become urgent.[11,22] Globally, women represent 43% of people infected by HIV/AIDS; more than 55% cent of people infected are in sub-Saharan Africa, 30% in Asia, and 20% in Europe and the United States (Population Council and International Family Health 2000).

AND THEY HAVE OTHER ADVANTAGES

Chemical barriers (microbicides) are a potential female-controlled method of STD prevention. However, even though numerous microbicide products are in development, the most optimistic estimates indicate that it will be a number of years before a microbicide is available. Moreover, the regulatory mechanisms necessary to approve microbicides could delay the use of a product once it is deemed safe and effective. Meanwhile, like others, we believe that the acceptability and STD-prevention efficacy of existing contraceptive methods must be investigated. The diaphragm is approved by the FDA and is available in the United States. Thus we argue that it is an excellent candidate for such research.

A microbicide—a compound that can be applied inside the vagina or rectum to protect against sexually transmitted infections—ultimately may be formulated as a gel, cream, film or suppository. An ideal microbicide should be effective, safe, acceptable, affordable, colourless, odourless, stable, easy to store and use, available in a variety of preparations, available in contraceptive and non-contraceptive formulations, and available without a prescription. At this time, however, the top priorities are to develop a microbicide that will provide protection when used consistently, and to develop a microbicide that will be used by those who need it most.[7]

It is important to support the development of microbicides because:

1. Diagnosis and treatment of STIs continues to spread, despite knowledge of successful HIV-prevention strategies.
2. Microbicides offer an alternative to condoms as a feasible means of primary prevention.
3. Currently available HIV-prevention techniques may not be feasible for many women in resource-poor settings.

In addition, microbicides are an option that women can use that may not require the cooperation of their partners. A recent cost-benefit analysis, conducted at the London School of Hygiene and Tropical Medicine, indicated that introducing a microbicide that reduces infection by 40% at 30% coverage could avert approximately six million HIV infections among men, women, and children in 73 lower-income countries.

References

1. Baume C A 2000 The relationship of perceived risk to condom use: why results are inconsistent. Soc Mar Q 6(1): 33–42
2. Closing the condom gap. Population reports Series H number 9 April 1999. Available at: www.jhuccp.org/pr/h9edsum.stm
3. Cody M M 1998 New developments in contraception: what's happening. Review. Clin Excell Nurse Pract 2(3):146–151
4. Condoms 1997 AIDS action. Mar–Aug(36–37):16–17
5. Elias C J et al 1996 Women-controlled HIV prevention methods. In: Mann J, Tarantola D (eds) AIDS in the World 11: global dimensions, social roots, and responses. The Global AIDS Policy Coalition. Oxford University Press, New York
6. Family Health International (FHI) 2000 How effective are spermicides? Network 20(2):11–15. Available online at www.fhi.org/en/fp/fppubs/network/v20–2/nt2022.html
7. Family Health International (FHI) 2000 Female barrier methods. Network 20(2). Available online at: www.fhi.org/en/fp/fppubs/network/v202/index.html
8. Feldblum P, Joanis C 1994 Modern barrier methods: effective contraception and diseases prevention. Family Health International
9. Femcap in Germany 2000 Contraceptive Technology Update 21(3):35–36
10. French P P et al 2003 Use effectiveness of the female versus male condom in preventing sexually transmitted diseases in women. Sexually Transmitted Diseases 30(5):433–439
11. Future contraceptive methods 1994 Contraceptive Reports 5(4):4–12
12. Gallo M F, Grimes D A, Schulz K F 2003 Non-latex versus latex male condoms for contraception. Review. Cochrane Database Systems Review 2:CD003550
13. Gallo M F et al 2003 Non-latex vs latex male condoms for contraception: a systemic review of randomized controlled trials. Contraception 68(5):319–326
14. Gilmour E 1996 Nonoxynol-9 and women's struggle against HIV. AIDS Anal Afr 6(5):14
15. How to use a female condom 1997 AIDS Action. Mar–Aug(36–37):17
16. How to use the diaphragm 1994 Contracep Rep 5(4):1–2
17. International Planned Parenthood Federation (IPPF) 1998 Medical Advisory Panel (IMAP) statement on the female condom. IPPF Medical Bulletin 32(3):
18. International Planned Parenthood Federation (IPPF) 2003 Medical Advisory Panel (IMAP) recommendations on nonoxynol-9. IPPF Medical Bulletin 37(1):2
19. International Planned Parenthood Federation (IPPF) 2000 Re-use of the female condom. IPPF Medical Bulletin 34(4). Available at www.ippf.org/medical/bulletin/pdf/e0008.pdf
20. Kuyoh M A et al 2003 Sponge versus diaphragm for contraception. (Cochrane Review) Cochrane Library, Issue 2. Update Software, Oxford
21. Lech M M 2002 Spermicides 2002: an overview. European Journal of Contraception and Reproduction Health Care 7(3):173–177
22. Lerner S Microbicides: a woman-controlled HIV prevention method in the making.
23. Lisken L et al 1990 Condoms now more than ever. Population Reports Series H, Number 8
24. Mauck C, Lai J J, Schwartz J, Weiner D H 2004 Diaphragms in clinical trials: is clinician fitting necessary? Contraception 24(4):263–266
25. Mishra S 1997 The female condom: expanding contraceptive options. Manushi Mar–Apr(99):37–38
26. Moench T et al 2001 Preventing disease by protecting the cervix: the unexplored promise of internal vaginal barrier devices. AIDS 15(13):1595–1602
27. National Institute of Allergy and Infectious Diseases (NIAID), National Institutes of Health (NIH), Department of Health and

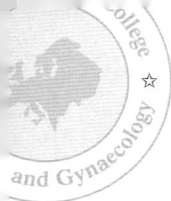

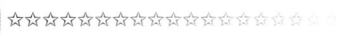

Human Services (DHHS) 2001 Scientific evidence on condom effectiveness for sexually transmitted diseases (STD) prevention: summary of workshop held June 12–13, 2000. Available at: www.niaid.nih.gov/dmid/stds/condomreport.pdf

28. 1995 New advantage 24 contraceptive gel claims 24-hour effectiveness, but proposed FDA rule could put N-9 products to the test. Contraceptive Technology Update 16(4):45–49

29. 1995 New data found on failure rates for female condoms. Rates similar to those of other barrier methods. Contraceptive Technology Update 16(4):54–55

30. PATH (Program for Appropriate Technology in Health) 1994 Condoms protect against STDs and HIV: correct and consistent use is key. Outlook 12(4)

31. PATH (Program for Appropriate Technology in Health) 2003 Re-examining the role of cervical barrier devices. Outlook 20(2):1–8. Available at www.path.org/files/eo120 2.pdf

32. PATH (Program for Appropriate Technology in Health) 1997 The female condom: for men and women. Outlook 15(4):1–8

33. PATH (Program for Appropriate Technology in Health) 1993 Vaginal barrier methods: underutilized options? Outlook 11(4)

34. POPLINE Digital Services. Condoms web site. Available at http:/condoms.jhucep.org/ [Accessed March 2003]

35. Raymond E G, Chen P L, Luoto J, Spermicide Trial Group 2004 Contraceptive effectiveness and safety of five nonoxynol-9 spermicides: a randomized trial. Obstetrics and Gynecology 103(3):430–439

36. SIECUS Report 1994 Jun–Jul; 22(5):10–13

37. 1993 Silicone rubber Femcap proves desirable to women. Contraception Technology Update 14(5):78–80

38. Steiner M J et al 2003 Contraceptive effectiveness of a polyurethane condom and a latex condom: a randomized controlled trial. Obstetrics and Gynecology 101(3):539–547

39. 1996 The cervical cap. Patient Update 4. Contraception Reports 7(4 Suppl):1–2

40. Wash N 1992 Alan Guttmacher Institute. Dec 21(20):1–2

41. WHO 2002 Considerations regarding reuses of the female condom: information update. Reproductive Health Matters 10(20):182–186

42. WHO, UNAIDS 2000 Consultation on the reuse of the female condom: information update (July). Available at: www.who.int/reproductive health/rtis/consultation on re-use of female condom Durban, en, html

43. WHO, UNAIDS Female Health Company The female condom: a guide for planning and programming. WHO/UNAIDS, Geneva. Available at: www.femalehealth.com/download/JC301-FemCondGuide-E.pdf

44. WHO, UNAIDS 2001 Effectiveness of condoms in preventing sexually transmitted infections including HIV. WHO/UNAIDS Information Note

45. WHO 2000 Effectiveness of male latex condoms in protecting against pregnancy and sexually transmitted infections. WHO Fact Sheet No 243. WHO, Geneva. Available at: www.who.int/reproductive-health/rtis/male condom.html

46. WHO 1997 The female condom: a review. WHO/HRP/WOM/97,1. WHO, Geneva

6

☆☆☆☆☆☆☆☆☆☆☆☆☆☆☆☆☆☆☆ ☆

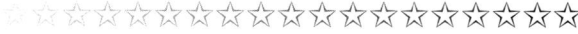

Progestogen-only methods of contraception

Anne Bachelot   Frédérique Kuttenn

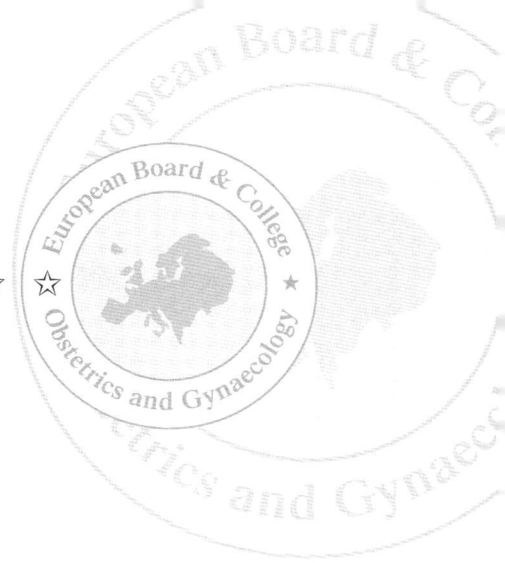

ABSTRACT

There are different types of progestogen-only methods of contraception, which are dependent on the dose and route of administration. Progestogen contraceptives include low-dose continuously administered or high-dose sequentially administered progestogens, long-acting injectable progestogens, implants, progestogen intrauterine devices, and continuous or intermittent vaginal rings. Progestins can also be used as emergency postcoital contraception. The mechanism of contraceptive action depends on the dose of progestogen administered. One of the mechanisms of action is a local effect, progestogens induce the formation of thick, viscid cervical mucus, altering motility of the Fallopian tube and reversibly suppressing endometrial development. Some of the progestogens have also been shown to interact with ovulation under certain methods of administration. They prevent ovulation by suppressing follicle-stimulating hormone (FSH) and luteinising hormone (LH) secretion. They also inhibit hypothalamic gonadotrophin-releasing hormone (GnRH) release and may have a direct effect on the pituitary.

Progestogen-only contraception offers a wide variety of methods, which constitute second-line contraception for the metabolic, vascular or cellular contraindications of estrogen-progestogen contraception, and permit various solutions to individual situations.

KEYWORDS

Contraception, progestogen, breast, progestin pills, injectable progestogens, progestogen implants, intrauterine, cervical vaginal rings, post-coital contraception

Contraception and family planning

INTRODUCTION

There is an increasing number of alternatives to combined oral contraceptives (COCs) intended for women who have metabolic, vascular or cellular contra-indications to COCs.

Progestogen contraceptives, including low-dose continuously administered or high-dose sequentially administered progestogens, long-acting injectable progestogens, implants, progestogen intrauterine devices, and continuous or discontinuous vaginal rings, are alternative progestogen contraceptive methods.

The progestogen used, the route of administration, the dose and duration of action, and especially the mechanisms of action, differ from one method to another. This variety offers a wide choice.

Some methods act only peripherally to change the consistency of cervical mucus, alter the endometrium, and reduce Fallopian tubal mobility, and do not affect hypothalamo–pituitary gonadotrophic function. Others inhibit ovulation. Some have preferential peripheral targets, but also have at least a partial antigonadotrophic action.

Progestogen methods have been evaluated for efficacy and some are slightly less effective than estrogen-progestogen pills. The hormonal profile and more specifically the FSH/LH balance and its consequences on the ovaries, and the estradiol/progesterone balance, which is essential for the target organs, uterus and breast, have not always been evaluated as meticulously as necessary. They may raise questions and need special attention in the future.

CLASSIFICATION

The progestogens used for contraception are synthetic. They are classified by structure: derivatives of 19-nortestosterone, 19-norprogesterone or 17-hydroxy-progesterone. The newest third-generation progestogens (desogestrel, norgestimate, and gestodene) are all derivatives of norgestrel and are also used in combination with ethinyl-estradiol for contraception.

Currently available progestogens interact with the progesterone receptor and with other steroid hormone receptors, including the androgen, glucocorticoid, mineralocorticoid and estrogen receptors. According to their specific profile, these molecules will exert actions other than the expected progestational activity.

MECHANISMS OF ACTION

The mechanism of contraceptive action depends on the dose of progestogen administered. One of the mechanisms of action is a local effect. Progestogens induce the formation of thick, viscid cervical mucus, which limits the penetrability of sperm; they alter motility of the Fallopian tube and reversibly suppress endometrial development, rendering it unsuitable for implantation. Some of the progestogens have also been shown to interact with ovulation under certain administration procedures. They prevent ovulation by suppression of follicle-stimulating hormone (FSH) and luteinising hormone (LH) secretion. They inhibit hypothalamic gonadotrophin-releasing hormone (GnRH) release and may also have a direct effect on the pituitary.

METHODS

There are different types of progestogen-only methods, depending on the dose and the route of administration. Progestins can be given orally, at low dose continuously, or at high dose discontinuously. There are injectable progestogens (depot medroxyprogesterone acetate and norethisterone enanthate), progestogen implants (such as Norplant®, Jadelle® and Implanon®), progesterone or levonorgestrel intrauterine devices and cervical vaginal rings. Progestogens can also be used as emergency postcoital contraception.

PROGESTIN-ONLY PILLS

LOW-DOSE PROGESTIN PILLS (POPs)

Current oral progestin-only formulations contain low doses of either norgestrienone (350 μg 24 h^{-1}), norethisterone acetate (600 μg 24 h^{-1}), levonorgestrel (30 μg 24 h^{-1}), lynestrenol (500 μg 24 h^{-1}) or desogestrel (75 μg 24 h^{-1}).

POPs appear to prevent conception through various combinations of these mechanisms, with great inter- and intra-individual variations. The effect of progestins on cervical mucus is the most immediate but shortest effect of protection provided by POPs, thereby serving as the first line of defence but offering full protection for less than 24 hours. This effect results in production of hostile, blocked mucus, and reduction of the volume of cervical mucus produced at midcycle, resulting in poor sperm penetration. Other mechanisms involved are the reduction in the number and size of endometrial glands, inhibition of progesterone receptor synthesis in the endometrium, preventing implantation and the reduction in the activity of the cilia in the Fallopian tube.[31] These peripheral effects are the principal mechanisms of action of POPs, but it is believed that some of these progestogen pills have systemic endocrinologic effects that interfere with ovulation by suppressing the LH surge. Nevertheless, basal secretion of FSH is preserved as well as partial follicular maturation and women may show persistent follicles or cysts.

POPs should be started on the first day of menses. If they are started later, a backup method should be used for the first 48 hours. Based on endogenous hormonal levels in the post-partum period, POPs should be initiated at three weeks for partial or non-breastfeeders, but can be delayed until three months postpartum for fully breastfeeding mothers, unless menses start before that time. POPs can and should be initiated immediately after an abortion.[31]

Plasma progestogen levels peak about two hours after oral administration, followed by rapid distribution and elimination. Plasma levels return to baseline values within 24 hours, making efficacy dependent upon rigid adherence to the dosing schedule.[31] There are large variations among individual users in plasma levels. The progestogen-only pill must then be taken continuously, regardless of bleeding patterns, at exactly the same time each day. Delay of more than three hours can lead to loss of contraceptive efficacy.

All these pills used worldwide are roughly equal in contraceptive effectiveness, with failure rates ranging from 1 to 2 per 100 woman-years, which rate is higher than with the combined estrogen-progestogen contraceptive pill.[24]

Progestin-only contraceptives are more effective in preventing intrauterine than ectopic pregnancies.[36] Thus, among progestin-only contraceptive failures the ratio of ectopic to intrauterine pregnancy is higher than in women who are not receiving oral contraceptives. This is due to alteration and slowing of Fallopian tubal motility. Moreover, diagnosis can be delayed because of common menstrual irregularity.

Masculinisation of female fetuses or hypospadias in male fetuses have not been reported as a result of low-dose progestin pill failure, most likely because of the small amounts of progestin in the formulations.[1]

The most common side effect is menstrual irregularity due to anovulation or dysovulation in 50% of cases, with erratic cycles and ovarian cysts. These drugs have found limited acceptance due to problems with irregular vaginal bleeding. Some women become amenorrhoeic, due to gonadotrophic interference, anovulation, loss of cyclic function and possibly endometrial atrophy.

It appears that the prevalence of headache, breast tenderness and, less often, nausea and dizziness may be slightly elevated among POP users. Androgenic side effects such as acne, hirsutism, and weight gain occur rarely.[31]

Low-dose progestin-only pills have only negligible effects on lipid metabolism.[6] Levels of cholesterol, LDL and VLDL are not affected by POP use. There is a suggestion of smaller decrease in HDL-cholesterol with the desogestrel-containing POP than with the levonorgestrel-containing POP and a significant difference between the two treatments for lipoprotein (a), but these changes are very small and not found in all studies. There is a trend towards higher glucose and insulin values with these pills, but none of the changes are clinically relevant. These progestogen-only pills have little effect on HbA_1C values[28] and little or no effect on coagulation factors;[47] they do not increase the prevalence of hypertension and do not appear to increase the risk of cardiovascular disease.

Accelerated metabolism of progestin pills has been reported with concurrent use of drugs such as rifampicin or enzyme-inducing anticonvulsant medications that induce microsomal liver enzymes.[31] These drugs should not be used with progestin pills, because they decrease their efficacy, with a risk of intrauterine or ectopic pregnancy.

Recently, POPs containing desogestrel were developed, based on the concept of a more potent ovulation inhibition than with other POPs. Studies have shown that desogestrel administered at a dose of $75\,\mu g\,d^{-1}$ has a greater effect on the inhibition of ovulation, suggesting that it would be more effective than other low-dose progestin pills.[12] The decrease in LH observed is significantly greater than with other low-dose progestin pills, indicating that the suppression of hypothalamic–pituitary axis is more pronounced. Nevertheless, no change was found in FSH levels, and women presented persistent follicles or cysts. Using the 90-day reference period for assessing the bleeding pattern, desogestrel users had a higher incidence of amenorrhoea and infrequent bleeding on the one hand, and of frequent bleeding and prolonged bleeding on the other hand, at the beginning of the study period. In contrast to the use of levonorgestrel, a tendency towards less bleeding over time was observed with the use of desogestrel.[38]

Contraception with low-dose progestin pills should therefore be reserved for women with high metabolic and vascular risk. In women with diabetes mellitus, hypertension, dyslipidaemia, and thromboembolic disease, combined estrogen-progestogen pills and even high-dose progestins are contraindicated, and POPs are a good alternative. They may also be useful for lactating women, since they have no significant effect on lactation.[39] The amount transferred to infants of lactating mothers is negligible.

However, since these pills do not have a strong antigonadotrophic action, they should not be given in cases of luteal insufficiency, polycystic ovary, endometrial hyperplasia, breast fibroadenoma, ovarian functional cysts and all hyperestrogenic states or unopposed estrogen situations. In these cases, high-dose progestins should be preferred.

HIGH-DOSE PROGESTIN PILLS

This therapeutic approach is based on the antigonadotrophic activity of progestins at high doses, associated with their peripheral effect. It is important to note that these high-dose progestin pills are not recommended by WHO for contraception, since the Pearl index has not been calculated.

19-nortestosterone derivatives

Current oral progestin formulations used for contraception are norgestrel, norethisterone acetate, etynodiol acetate, lynestrenol and norethynodrel. The 19-nortestosterone derivatives have a high affinity for the progesterone receptor, and have been shown to bind partly to the androgen receptor. Norgestrel has the most powerful progestogen and antigonadotrophic action, but it is associated with a mild androgenic activity. The other compounds (norethisterone acetate, etynodiol acetate, lynestrenol, norethynodrel) are partly metabolised to norethisterone.

Administration should be done for 21 days, from day 5 to day 25 of the cycle, or for 16 days, from day 10 to day 25 of the cycle, to induce an antigonadotrophic effect.[16] It has been shown that oral administration of lynestrenol 10 mg d^{-1} for 16 or 21 days induces antigonadotrophic activity, with low gonadotrophin levels and suppression of ovulation.[30] Administration for 16 days does not suppress endometrial development and then does not lead to amenorrhoea.

This contraception method may have several adverse effects, such as minor symptoms of hyperandrogenicity, acne and seborrhoea. High doses (10–40 mg d^{-1}) of norethisterone administered in early pregnancy may cause masculinisation of the female fetus, as well as hypospadias in male fetuses,[1] however, the individual risk is small. Less is known about the virilisation potential of other 19-nortestosterone derivatives, although similar effects could be expected at high doses. Metabolic adverse effects are observed with 19-nortestosterone derivatives, such as weight gain and insulin-resistance.[8] In predisposed women, they can lead to diabetes mellitus. A decrease in high-density lipoprotein (HDL) level, probably due to activation of hepatic lipase activity, has also been reported. These effects are related to the androgenic activity, dose, and route of administration of the progestins, while low-dose progestin-only pills and injectable progestins have little or no effect on lipoprotein levels. This can lead to a deleterious vascular effect. Nevertheless, no epidemiological study has evaluated the cardiovascular risk of high-dose progestogen pills. However, no change in blood pressure or coagulation factors (except for lynestrenol, which decreases antithrombin III levels) have been reported with these treatments.[13] Taken as described, these progestogens lead to hypoestrogenia, with unknown bone and vascular long-term effects.

Because of these metabolic effects, these high-dose progestogen pills are contraindicated in cases of obesity, diabetes mellitus, thromboembolic antecedent and hypertension.

These progestogens can be used for second-choice contraception. They are mostly administered for 21 days per cycle, and sometimes proposed for only 16 days per cycle (from the 10th to the 25th day of the cycle) in women who have long menstrual cycles with late or no ovulation.[30] They should be reserved for women who take advantage of hypoestrogeny because of benign breast or endometrial disease. They can be very useful in women who suffer from unopposed estrogen situations, such as endometrial hyperplasia, fibroadenoma or fibrocystic breast disease, and functional ovarian cysts.

17-hydroxyprogesterone and 19-norprogesterone derivatives

The principal molecules derived from 17-hydroxyprogesterone and used for contraception are chlormadinone acetate, medrogestone, medroxyprogesterone acetate, and cyproterone acetate. These derivatives of 17-hydroxyprogesterone have a high affinity for the progesterone receptor, do not exert androgenic or metabolic side effects and have limited antigonadotrophic activity compared with derivatives of 19-nortestosterone.[37] The mechanisms of action of these progestogens are different: chlormadinone acetate, medrogestone and medroxyprogesterone acetate have luteomimetic and antigonadotrophic activity, whereas cyproterone acetate has antigonadotrophic and antiandrogenic effects.

Demegestone, promegestone and nomegestrol acetate are derivatives of 19-norprogesterone. They bind progesterone receptors with a high affinity, but have little or no affinity for the estrogen, androgen and aldosterone receptors. Some authors have proposed the use of chlormadinone acetate (10 mg d^{-1}), promegestone (500 µg d^{-1}) and nomegestrol acetate (5 mg d^{-1}) for 21 days, from day 5 to day 25 of the cycle, as contraception. It is important to note the potent antigonadotrophic activity and ovulation inhibition of these compounds shown in these studies.[5,7,16,17] Nevertheless, further studies are needed to confirm the efficacy of these derivatives in contraception.

These compounds seem to have very limited deleterious metabolic effects. Their oral administration does not appear to affect blood pressure, coagulation factors, lipoproteins, insulinaemia or carbohydrate tolerance. Derivatives of

19-norprogesterone and 17-hydroxyprogesterone do not appear to increase the risk of stroke or venous thromboembolism.[13,14] Nevertheless, additional studies are needed to evaluate those effects. One side effect is menstrual irregularity or amenorrhoea, but the incidence of menstrual disorders has not been fully evaluated. When administered for 20 days per 28, these progestogens may lead to hypoestrogenia, with unevaluated bone and vascular effects.

Administration for 21 days should be reserved as second-choice contraception in women with a contraindication to combined oral contraceptives, or in women who suffer from unopposed estrogen situations, such as endometrial or benign breast disease, ovarian functional cysts, or who have vascular or metabolic contraindications to 19-nortestosterone derivatives.

These high-dose progestin pills have other non-contraceptive benefits, such as regulation of menstrual dysfunction. They also have long been used for the treatment of symptoms associated with endometriosis.[44] Although this approach to therapy has been superseded by the development of danazol and GnRH analogues, progestins are still useful for the long-term treatment of patients with symptomatic endometriosis who wish to preserve future fertility but are not actively attempting pregnancy. 17-Hydroxyprogesterone and 19-norprogesterone derivatives can also be useful in pathologic conditions such as systemic diseases that can take advantage of hypoestrogeny, such as SLE (systemic lupus erythematous).[27] In such a disease, pure progestogen contraception seems to be antigonadotrophic and anti-estrogenic enough and devoid of metabolic or vascular side effects, whereas norsteroid progestogens may have metabolic side effects and low-dose progestogen pills tend to induce cystic ovaries and high plasma estradiol levels.

LONG-ACTING CONTRACEPTIVE STEROIDS

A variety of long-acting steroid contraceptives have been developed as alternatives to oral agents. Originally, they were developed to eliminate the estrogen component of oral contraceptives. The primary advantage of this contraception is that efficacy does not depend on patient compliance.

INJECTABLE STEROIDS

The principle. Long-acting injectable progestogen contraceptives are depot medroxyprogesterone acetate (DMPA, 150 mg IM every three months) and norethindrone enanthate (200 mg IM every eight weeks for six months, and then every 12 weeks). A number of progestogens are being tested as long-acting injectable agents in the form of microspheres or microcapsules that release hormones slowly at a constant rate and are effective for 1–6 months.

Depot medroxyprogesterone acetate

Depot medroxyprogesterone acetate (DMPA) is the only injectable contraceptive approved for use in the USA. It is the long-acting formulation of medroxyprogesterone acetate and consists of a crystalline suspension of this hormone. MPA

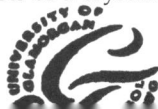

can be detected in the systemic circulation within 30 minutes after intramuscular injection.[35] Although plasma MPA levels vary between individuals, they rise steadily to contraceptively effective plasma levels (>0.5 ng ml^{-1}) within 24 hours after injection, and are maintained at approximately 1 ng ml^{-1} for three months. MPA remains detectable in the circulation (>0.2 ng ml^{-1}) for 7–9 months.[35]

The major mechanism of action of DMPA is inhibition of ovulation. It also induces the production of a thick, unfavourable cervical mucus so sperm are unlikely to reach the oviduct and fertilise the ovocyte, and a decidual reaction, which results in an unfavourable endometrium, and it may delay Fallopian ovum transport. Histological examination of endometrial biopsy in women who received MPA revealed three types of pattern: proliferative, quiescent, and atrophic.

To obtain suppression of ovulation in the initial injection cycle, DMPA has to be administered within a few days after the onset of menses, before day 5 of the cycle. Estradiol levels are found to be in the range of the early follicular to mid-follicular phase but below 100 pg ml^{-1} during the first two months after injection, and show a significant rise at the end of the 12-week period.[11,26,33,40] Although the midcycle LH peak is suppressed after the injection, tonic LH is still being secreted in a pulsatile manner, and the levels are about the same as those found in the follicular phase of the control cycle.[33] The normally occurring peak level of FSH at midcycle is also suppressed after the injection, but tonic FSH levels are in the range of those found in the follicular phase, indicating a lack of complete suppression of the hypothalamic–pituitary axis. After 4–6 months, when MPA levels decrease to less than 0.5 ng ml^{-1}, plasma estradiol rises to preovulatory levels, indicating follicular activity, but ovulation does not occur, as evidenced by low progesterone levels.[11,33,40] Return of follicular activity precedes the return of luteal activity within 2–3 months. The return of luteal activity occurs 7–9 months after the injection, when MPA levels are below 0.1 ng ml^{-1}.[11,33,40] Because of the prolonged clearing time of DMPA from the circulation, resumption of ovulation may be delayed for up to one year after the last injection. Women who stop using DMPA to become pregnant should be informed that the resumption of fertility will be delayed until the drug is cleared from the circulation.

DMPA is an effective contraceptive. In a large clinical trial on DMPA use, the pregnancy rate at one year was only 0.1%. At two years, the cumulative rate was 0.4%.[48] The failure rates are lower than with the estrogen-progestogen combined pill. Benefits include good compliance, a fivefold reduction in the risk of endometrial carcinoma and no overall increased risk of breast, cervical, endometrial or ovarian cancer.

Several side effects may be associated with this method. The most common include irregular uterine bleeding and spotting. In the first three months after the first injection, about 30% of women are amenorrhoeic and another 30% have irregular bleeding and spotting occurring more than 11 days per month.[40] Bleeding is due to atrophy during the first weeks after the injection, when estradiol levels are low, and endometrial hyperplasia at the end of the 12-week period, when estradiol levels rise. The bleeding is usually small in amount and does not cause anaemia. As duration of therapy increases, the incidence of frequent bleeding steadily declines,

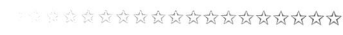

and the incidence of amenorrhoea steadily increases, so that by the end of two years about 70% of the women treated with DMPA are amenorrhoeic. Other side effects include weight gain and depression. DMPA has several metabolic effects.[46] It decreases HDL-cholesterol levels, increases LDL-cholesterol levels, and stimulates the appetite in the early months of use, which can lead to weight gain. This effect diminishes with longer use.

DMPA has partial androgenic and glucocorticoid effects, however it does not seem to modify glucose or insulin levels.[46] It has not been associated with an increased incidence of hypertension or thromboembolism. Nevertheless, its contraindications include active thrombophlebitis, current or past history of thromboembolic disorders, current or past history of cerebral vascular disease, liver dysfunction and known or suspected malignancy of the breast.

Norethindrone enanthate

Norethindrone enanthate has a shorter duration of action and is less effective than medroxyprogesterone acetate.[48] Pregnancy rates are slightly higher with norethindrone enanthate than with medroxyprogesterone acetate. The pregnancy rates with both treatment methods are higher shortly after the first injection.

Long-acting injectable contraceptives should be reserved for women in developing countries or for women who comply poorly to oral contraception. Women with psychiatric illness and those who are mentally handicapped also may benefit from the convenience associated with the use of injectable contraceptives.

IMPLANTS

Norplant® and Jadelle®

Subdermal implantation of polydimethysiloxone (Silastic®) capsules or rods containing a variety of progestogens has been used for contraception. Various progestins have been investigated, and by 1974 the six-capsule Silastic® drug-delivery system, which was to become the Norplant® contraceptive system, was made ready for clinical trials.

Norplant® implant is an effective, reversible, long-term method of fertility regulation that has particular advantages for women who wish to have an extended period of contraceptive protection. The system consists of six, soft, flexible capsules of Silastic® rubber that contain levonorgestrel.

The capsules are inserted in a superficial plane beneath the skin on the inside of the upper arm and must be removed after the steroid has been released. To ensure that the woman is not pregnant at the time of capsule placement and to ensure contraceptive effectiveness during the first cycle of use, it is advisable that insertion be done during the first seven days of the menstrual cycle, or immediately following an abortion. Insertion is not recommended before six weeks of postpartum in breastfeeding women.[21] Once in place, levonorgestrel provides effective protection against pregnancy during the first month and through five years of use. Immediately after implantation, the dose of levonorgestrel provided by Norplant® implants is about $85\,\mu g\,d^{-1}$. This declines to about $50\,\mu g\,d^{-1}$ by nine months, to about $35\,\mu g\,d^{-1}$ by 18 months, and to about $30\,\mu g\,d^{-1}$ over the remaining five years of use.[18] The plasma levonorgestrel levels achieved as this progestin diffuses out of the Silastic® capsules are lower than those usually observed in women using oral combined estrogen-progestogen contraceptives containing 100–150 μg of levonorgestrel. However, the greater effectiveness of the implants relates to the constancy of the plasma levels rather than the peaks and valleys that occur after the use of each pill. The concentrations of levonorgestrel in women show considerable variation, depending on body weight and individual clearance rates. Nonetheless, individual levels remain relatively constant.

Norplant® implants therefore mediate their effects on fertility by a variety of mechanisms, including alteration of cervical mucus, and suppression of endometrium development, which becomes unsuitable for implantation. Examination of cervical mucus from Norplant® implant users shows that most women have scanty mucus that is extremely viscid, and thus sperm penetration is impaired and fertilisation cannot occur.

Another mechanism of action of Norplant® is its interaction with ovulation. Every-other-day blood samples from a randomly selected group of users have shown plasma progesterone levels compatible with ovulation in some women. Furthermore, the percentage of women with elevated serum progesterone levels suggestive of ovulation increases with longer durations of Norplant® implant use. After 3–5 years, approximately 50% of women using implants have plasma progesterone levels consistent with ovulation. Thus, ovulation suppression does not entirely account for this method's effectiveness. In some users, the mid-cycle surges of LH are blunted even though cyclic ovarian estradiol secretion by the ovary continues. Ultrasonic studies show that many women who have regular menses while using Norplant® implants develop a follicle that does not rupture but regresses over several weeks.

During the first year of use, only 0.2% of all continuing users became pregnant. In the second year, the pregnancy rate was 0.5% for all users. During years three to five, the pregnancy rates rose to over 1% per year. After two years of use, differences in pregnancy rates were noted among women of different weights. For example, in women less than 50 kg, there were almost no pregnancies, even after five years of use, while in women heavier than 70 kg, the yearly pregnancy rate rose to 2.5–5.1% in years three and four. When implants were used for longer than five years, the annual pregnancy rate rose to 2.5–3.0% for all users. Therefore Norplant® implants should be replaced at the end of five years.

Norplant® has several adverse effects. Bruising may occur at the implant site during insertion or removal. Other cutaneous reactions that have been reported include blistering, ulcerations, and sloughing. There have been reports of arm pain, numbness, and tingling following these procedures. In some women, hyperpigmentation occurs over the implantation site but is usually reversible following removal. There have been reports of capsule displacement, most of which involve minor changes in the positioning of the capsules.

The major reason women stop using Norplant® implants is menstrual irregularity similar to that associated with oral low-dose progestin pills.[15] Menometrorrhagia is the prime reason for terminating implant use. Nevertheless, it has been shown that menstrual flow volume decreases during implant use. The total number of bleeding days per year declines significantly from a mean of 54 days per year in year one to 44 days in year five. The total number of spotting days per year also decreases significantly after the first year. Disruption of the normal cycle during implant use produces long intervals without frank bleeding, although spotting often occurs in such intervals. Mood changes and headache also may lead to discontinuation.

Functional ovarian cysts and delayed follicular atresia develop in some women using Norplant® implants.[3] These cysts, some of which are 7–10 cm in diameter, regress over several weeks. Because, to the casual examiner, enlarged follicles may be indistinguishable from ovarian cysts due to other causes, women using Norplant® implants and their health-care providers should be advised that usually functional ovarian cysts occur and that invasive measures are not required. The incidence of ovarian cysts requiring surgery is not greater than that in women who do not use hormonal contraception.

Another medical reason for terminating Norplant® implant use is infection at the site of insertion. This rare event (0.7% of users) is usually associated with inadequate asepsis and no longer occurs once health-care providers gain experience.

Some drugs, such as rifampicin or enzyme-inducing anticonvulsants, increase the risk of pregnancy in implant users because they increase the rate of levonorgestrel metabolism. Evidence of drug interaction is the most convincing in the case of phenytoin and carbamazepine.

Ectopic pregnancies have occurred among users of Norplant® capsules at an average rate of 1.3 per 1000 woman-years. The risk of ectopic pregnancy may increase with time, with duration of use, and possibly with weight. Thus, implants must be replaced after five years.

Implants appear to induce mild insulin resistance but no significant change in serum glucose levels.[22] Changes from baseline in the lipid and apolipoprotein parameters tested were generally not significant.[42] Until greater experience is available, clinical judgment and experience with other hormonal contraceptives suggest that Norplant® implants should not be used in women with active thrombophlebitis or thromboembolic disorders, undiagnosed abnormal genital bleeding, known or suspected pregnancy, acute liver disease, benign or malignant liver tumours, known or suspected carcinoma of the breast, history of idiopathic intracranial hypertension, or hypersensitivity to levonorgestrel or any of the components of the Norplant® implants.

Thus, a major advantage of this contraceptive is that the efficacy of Norplant® implants does not depend on patient compliance. The effects of Norplant® implants are reversible. Observations in women who terminated use because they desired to become pregnant suggest that later fecundity was not altered. The life table pregnancy rates were 24% at one month after removal, 90% at one year, and 95% at two years.

The Norplant® system, which consists of six implants, has recently been largely superseded by Jadelle®, which requires implantation of only two silicone-based polymer rods. Each rod is 43 mm in length and 2.5 mm in diameter and contains 75 mg of levonorgestrel. After insertion Jadelle® continuously releases levonorgestrel for five years. The mechanism of action is similar to that of the Norplant® system. One set of rods provides contraceptive protection for five years with pregnancy rates of 0–0.8% per year of use (1.1% over five years).

Implanon®

There is a new subdermal contraceptive implant containing a norsteroid progestin—etonogestrel (3 keto-desogestrel): Implanon® (Fig 6.1). It is a single-rod implant system. The manufacturer claims that the etonogestrel implant requires 1–2 minutes for insertion and removal and provides contraception for up to three years. The contraceptive efficacy of Implanon® is high, with zero pregnancies in 53 530 cycles (4103 woman-years), resulting in a Pearl index of 0.0 (95% CI: 0.00–0.09).[19]

Implanon® prevents pregnancy essentially by changing the character of the cervical mucus and the endometrium.[43] The resulting effects are characterised by alterations in endometrial histology, endometrial thickness, dysmenorrhoea and menstrual bleeding pattern. It interacts with ovulation, suppressing the midcycle peaks of LH, but does not interfere with FSH. Moreover, it is important to note that little is known about estradiol levels, follicular growth and incidence of ovarian cysts with Implanon®. Preliminary studies show that although it initially suppresses follicular development and estradiol production, ovarian activity slowly increases after six months, and FSH and estradiol levels are almost normal. Endogenous progesterone levels remain in the subovulatory range for >3 years in most women.[9]

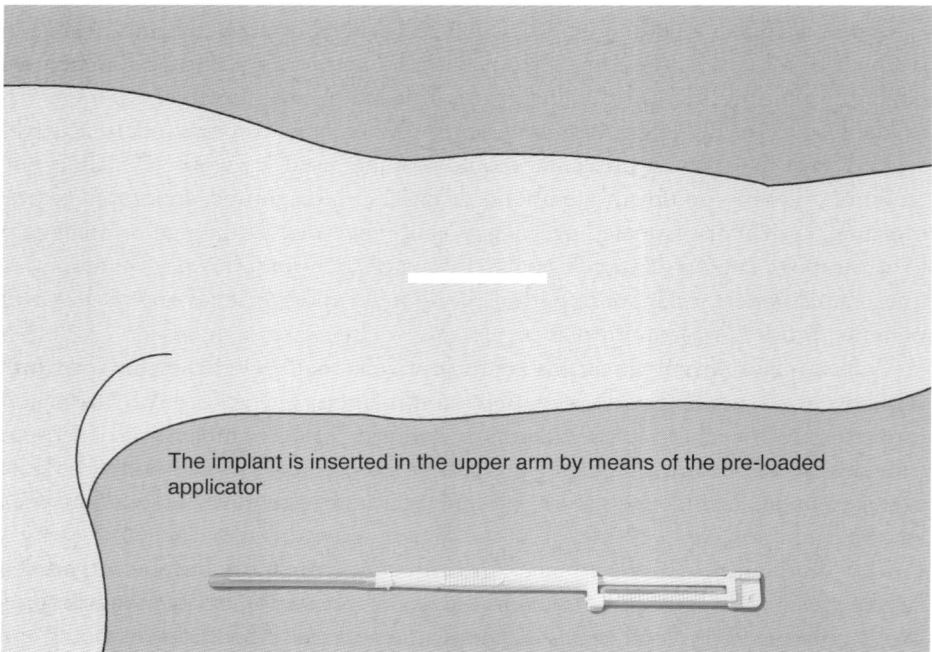

The implant is inserted in the upper arm by means of the pre-loaded applicator

Fig 6.1 The gestagen implant Implanon® and its applicator. (Courtesy of Organon AB)

Implanon® users had more amenorrhoea, slightly less frequent bleeding, and prolonged bleeding than Norplant® users.[2]

Although implants are effective, they need to be removed and are associated with amenorrhoea and breakthrough bleeding similar to that seen with oral low-dose progestin pills. They are well adapted to women in developing countries who desire effective hormonal contraception and do not want sterilisation. Women with psychiatric illness and those who are mentally handicapped may also benefit from the convenience associated with use of implantable contraceptives. This progestin-only birth control method can be used by lactating women.

INTRAUTERINE DEVICES

Progestin-releasing IUDs are described in Ch. 4.

CONTRACEPTIVE VAGINAL RINGS (CVRs)

Contraceptive vaginal rings (CVRs) contain sex steroids that diffuse through a plastic polymer ring at a constant rate and are absorbed directly through the vaginal epithelium into the systemic circulation. This delivery system provides many advantages over oral contraceptives (OCs), including avoidance of the first-pass effect through the liver, thus allowing for lower effective doses, providing constant plasma steroid levels, longer duration of use, and greater bioavailability of the hormones. Vaginal rings also have the advantage of being user-controlled and non-provider dependent, and their use is non-coital related. CVRs containing only progestin are designed either for 3–6 months continuous use, with a contraceptive effect due to a peripheral effect on cervical mucus, endometrium, and tubal motility, but with some interference with ovulation, or for discontinuous use, with a contraceptive effect due to inhibition of ovulation.

The first CVR to be studied released medroxyprogesterone acetate. Numerous clinical trials testing various steroids and doses have followed. Early progestin-only rings, which contained 100 mg of medroxyprogesterone acetate, successfully suppressed ovulation. They were removed after 21 days of use to allow withdrawal bleeding and were replaced on day five of the cycle.[32]

Early norgestrel rings provided excellent cycle inhibition.[34] The World Health Organization tested levonorgestrel-releasing vaginal rings extensively, culminating in a multinational trial of 20 μg levonorgestrel-releasing rings.[29] The rings were to be worn for three consecutive months by more than 1000 women. The devices were effective, with a 12-month pregnancy rate of 3.6 per 100 women. The primary reasons for discontinuation were menstrual disturbances (17.2 per 100 women at one year), followed by frequent expulsion of the ring (6.1 per 100 women), and vaginal epithelial lesions that halted further product development (6.0%). The finding of erythematous lesions in the vagina in some women has led to the development of a more flexible device. As with other progestin-only methods, menstrual blood loss was actually two-thirds of baseline.

The first published report in 1989 described ethylene vinyl acetate rings measuring 4 × 56 mm and releasing 15 or 30 μg of etonogestrel (ETG) per day. The pharmacokinetics of ring insertion and removal were assessed. No burst progestin release was seen. In the plateau phase, release rates decreased 5% per 21-day cycle.[25]

Other progestogens in CVRs which have been tested are norgestrienone, megestrol, and nestorone. Nestorone (ST-1435 or 17-acetoxy-16-methylene-19-norprogesterone) is a novel progestin with low androgenicity, which is being studied by the Population Council. The vaginal ring is made of Silastic® with a core containing 77 mg of nestorone and releasing $100 \mu g \, d^{-1}$. Nestorone has been tested alone in vaginal rings, used on a three weeks in/one week out regimen That experience showed that the nestorone ring had a high frequency of luteal activity, which occurred mostly after the one-week ring-free interval. This led to the conclusion that a progestin-only ring should be used continuously to be effective.[23] Continuous use was subsequently studied at the dose of $100 \mu g$. Plasma levels of nestorone achieved in CVR users were approximately 280 pmol L^{-1} at one month and 220 pmol L^{-1} at six months. The CVR users had a high incidence of amenorrhoea (47%) in the second three-month period and a decline in irregular bleeding/spotting from 81% in the first three months to 32% in the last three months. Frequent and prolonged bleeding/spotting patterns were absent in the last three months. Ovulation inhibition was achieved in over 97%.[10] The six-month cumulative pregnancy rate was 2.1%. Circulating estradiol levels ranged from 100 to 150 pg ml^{-1}. Nestorone is transformed to inactive metabolites when orally administered. Therefore this ring can be prescribed to breastfeeding women.

Vaginal rings of homogenous design with up to 2.2 mg of progesterone release per day and 0.22 mg of estradiol were evaluated in cycling women for thirty 21-day cycles to study the effect on ovarian function, but they demonstrated poor cycle control and unreliable ovulation inhibition.[45] A larger study using rings inserted in lactating women at day 60 postpartum and replaced every three months with a new one releasing 10 mg of progesterone alone found one pregnancy in 739 woman-months of use compared with 19 pregnancies in the 677 woman-months using lactation only.[20] Serum progesterone levels ranged from 33 nmol L^{-1} in the first week to 10 nmol L^{-1} in the 16th week of continuous use. These levels are within the range shown to inhibit fertility in lactating women. A multicentre study comparing a vaginal ring releasing 10 mg of progesterone daily with a copper intrauterine device in 1500 lactating women found a one-year pregnancy rate of 1.7 and 0.5%, respectively.[41] The commercial product was fabricated for three-months' continuous use with average daily release of 10 mg of progesterone. No pregnancy occurred during more than 1200 months of exposure with the vaginal ring. These rings are indicated for use in breastfeeding women.

CVRs have several adverse effects. Expulsion is rare, but is occasionally seen with bowel movements, straining, or tampon removal.[4] The size is a compromise. When a 50 mm ring was compared with a 58 mm ring, women experienced more expulsions with the smaller ring.

The vast majority of women do not remove the ring for intercourse. In a Latin American study, only 10% of women removed the ring for every sex act. Fewer than 1–2% experienced discomfort or reported discomfort from their partners. Some partners seemed unaware of the device. Less than 1% of women reported difficulties with odour that they attributed to the ring. All rings are associated with increased vaginal secretions. Vaginal discharge is one of the reason for discontinuation. The mechanical reaction stimulates some discharge because unmedicated rings show similar rates of discharge. The vaginal bacteriology of device users was similar to oral contraceptive users. A number of women have developed monolial vaginitis or bacterial vaginosis during use.[4] This type of contraception should be interrupted in cases of infection resistant to agent-specific anti-infectious treatment.

EMERGENCY POSTCOITAL CONTRACEPTION

Emergency postcoital contraception with progestins is described in Ch. 7.

CONCLUSION

Progestogen-only contraception offers a wide variety of methods, which constitute second-line contraceptions for the metabolic and vascular contraindications of estrogen-progestogen contraception, and permit various answers to individual situations. Special attention should be paid to the final estrogen-progestogen balance resulting from these treatments and its compatibility with the individual profile and the breast and endometrial status of these patients.

References

1. Aarskog D 1979 Maternal progestins as a possible cause of hypospadias. New England Journal of Medicine 300:75–78
2. Affandi B 1998 An integrated analysis of vaginal bleeding patterns in clinical trials of Implanon. Contraception 58(6 Suppl): 99S–107S
3. Alvarez-Sanchez F, Brache V, de Oca V M, Cochon L, Faundes A 2000 Prevalence of enlarged ovarian follicles among users of levonorgestrel subdermal contraceptive implants (Norplant). American Journal of Obstetrics and Gynecology 182:535–539
4. Ballagh S A 2001 Vaginal ring hormone delivery systems in contraception and menopause. Clinical Obstetrics and Gynecology 44:106–113
5. Basdevant A, Pelissier C, Conard J, Degrelle H, Guyene T T, Thomas J L 1991 Effects of nomegestrol acetate (5 mg/d) on hormonal, metabolic and hemostatic parameters in premenopausal women. Contraception 44:599–605
6. Barkfeldt J, Virkkunen A, Dieben T 2001 The effects of two progestogen-only pills containing either desogestrel (75 microg/day) or levonorgestrel (30 microg/day) on lipid metabolism. Contraception 64:295–299
7. Bazin B, Thevenot R, Bursaux C, Paris J 1987 Effect of nomegestrol acetate, a new 19-norprogesterone derivative, on pituitary–ovarian function in women. British Journal of Obstetrics and Gynaecology 94:1199–1204
8. Beck P 1977 Effect of progestins on glucose and lipid metabolism. Annals of the New York Academy of Sciences 286:434–445
9. Bennink H J 2000 The pharmacokinetics and pharmacodynamics of Implanon, a single-rod etonogestrel contraceptive implant. European Journal of Contraception and Reproductive Health Care 5(Suppl 2):12–20
10. Brache V, Mishell D R, Lahteenmaki P, Alvarez F, Elomaa K, Jackanicz T, Faundes A 2001 Ovarian function during use of vaginal rings delivering three different doses of Nestorone. Contraception 63:257–261
11. Clark M K, Sowers M, Levy B T, Tenhundfeld P 2001 Magnitude and variability of sequential estradiol and progesterone concentrations in women using depot medroxyprogesterone acetate for contraception. Fertility and Sterility 75:871–877

12. Collaborative Study Group on the Desogestrel-containing Progestogen-only Pill 1998 A double-blind study comparing the contraceptive efficacy, acceptability and safety of two progestogen-only pills containing desogestrel 75 micrograms/day or levonorgestrel 30 micrograms/day. European Journal of Contraception and Reproductive Health Care 3:169–178

13. Conard J, Plu-Bureau G, Bahi N, Horellou M H, Pelissier C, Thalabard J C 2004 Progestogen-only contraception in women at high risk of venous thromboembolism. Contraception 70:437–441

14. Conard J, Samama M 1983 The effects of progestins on coagulation. In: Bardin C W, Milgrom E, Mauvais-Jarvis P (eds) Progesterone and progestins. Raven Press, New York, pp 447–452

15. Coukell A J, Balfour J A 1998 Levonorgestrel subdermal implants. A review of contraceptive efficacy and acceptability. Drugs 55:861–887

16. Couzinet B, Young J, Brailly S, Chanson P, Thomas J L, Schaison G 1996 The antigonadotropic activity of progestins (19-nortestosterone and 19-norprogesterone derivatives) is not mediated through the androgen receptor. Journal of Clinical Endocrinology and Metabolism 81: 4218–4223

17. Couzinet B, Young J, Kujas M, Meduri G, Brailly S, Thomas J L, Chanson P, Schaison G 1999 The antigonadotropic activity of a 19-norprogesterone derivative is exerted both at the hypothalamic and pituitary levels in women. Journal of Clinical Endocrinology and Metabolism 84:4191–4196

18. Croxatto H B, Diaz S, Brandeis A, Pavez M, Johansson E D 1985 Plasma levonorgestrel and progesterone levels in women treated with Silastic covered rods containing levonorgestrel. Contraception 31:643–654

19. Croxatto H B, Makarainen L 1998 The pharmacodynamics and efficacy of Implanon. An overview of the data. Contraception 58(6 Suppl):91S–97S

20. Diaz S, Jackanicz T M, Herreros C, Juez G, Peralta O, Miranda P, Casado M E, Schiapacasse V, Salvatierra A M, Brandeis A et al 1985 Fertility regulation in nursing women: VIII. Progesterone plasma levels and contraceptive efficacy of a progesterone-releasing vaginal ring. Contraception 32:603–622

21. Diaz S 2002 Contraceptive implants and lactation. Contraception 65(1):39–46

22. Dorflinger L J 2002 Metabolic effects of implantable steroid contraceptives for women. Contraception 65:47–62

23. Fraser I S, Weisberg E, Minehan E, Johansson E D 2000 A detailed analysis of menstrual blood loss in women using Norplant and Nestorone progestogen-only contraceptive implants or vaginal rings. Contraception 61:241–251

24. Graham S, Fraser I S 1982 The progestogen-only mini-pill. Contraception 26:373–388

25. Jackson R, Newton J R 1989 Pharmacodynamics of a contraceptive vaginal ring releasing 3-keto-desogestrel. Contraception 39:653–664

26. Jeppsson S, Johansson E D, Ljungberg O, Sjoberg N O 1977 Endometrial histology and circulating levels of medroxyprogesterone acetate (MPA), estradiol, FSH and LH in women with MPA induced amenorrhoea compared with women with secondary amenorrhoea. Acta Obstetricia et Gynecologica Scandinavica 56:43–48

27. Jungers P, Liote F, Dehaine V, Dougados M, Viriot J, Pelissier C, Kuttenn F 1990 Hormonal contraception and lupus. Annales de Medecine Interne (Paris) 141:253–256

28. Kivela A, Ruuskanen M, Agren U, Dieben T 2001 The effects of two progestogen-only pills containing either desogestrel (75 microgram/day) or levonorgestrel (30 microgram/day) on carbohydrate metabolism and adrenal and thyroid function. The European Journal of Contraception & Reproductive Health Care 6:71–77

29. Koetsawang S, Ji G, Krishna U, Cuadros A, Dhall G I, Wyss R, Rodriquez la Puenta J, Andrade A T, Khan T, Kononova E S et al 1990 Microdose intravaginal levonorgestrel contraception: a multicentre clinical trial. I. Contraceptive efficacy and side effects. World Health Organization Task Force on Long-Acting Systemic Agents for Fertility Regulation. Contraception 41:105–124

30. Kuttenn F, Moufarege A, Mauvais-Jarvis P 1978 The hormonal basis of discontinuous progestational contraception. Nouvelle Presse Medicale 7:3109–3113

31. McCann M F, Potter L S 1994 Progestin-only oral contraception: a comprehensive review. Contraception 50(6 Suppl 1): S1–S195

32. Mishell D R Jr, Talas M, Parlow A F, Moyer D L 1970 Contraception by means of a Silastic vaginal ring impregnated with

medroxyprogesterone acetate. American Journal of Obstetrics and Gynecology 107:100–107

33. Mishell D R Jr, Kharma K M, Thorneycroft I H, Nakamura R M 1972 Estrogenic activity in women receiving an injectable progestogen for contraception. American Journal of Obstetrics and Gynecology 113:372–376

34. Mishell D R Jr, Lumkin M, Jackanicz T 1975 Initial clinical studies of intravaginal rings containing norethindrone and norgestrel. Contraception 12:253–260

35. Mishell D R Jr 1996 Pharmacokinetics of depot medroxyprogesterone acetate contraception. Journal of Reproductive Medicine 41(5 Suppl):381–390

36. Netter A 1996 Ectopic pregnancies in subjects on progestin-only pills. Fertility and Sterility 65:1078–1079

37. Pelissier C, Blacker C, Feinstein M C, Cournot A, Denis C 1994 Antiovulatory action of chlormadinone acetate. Contraception Fertilité Sexualité 22:37–40

38. Rice C, Killick S, Hickling D, Coelingh Bennink H 1996 Ovarian activity and vaginal bleeding patterns with a desogestrel-only preparation at three different doses. Human Reproduction 11:737–740

39. Saarikoski S 1993 Contraception during lactation. Annals of Medicine 25:181–184

40. Schwallie P C, Assenzo J R 1974 The effect of depo-medroxyprogesterone acetate on pituitary and ovarian function, and the return of fertility following its discontinuation: a review. Contraception 10:181–202

41. Sivin I, Diaz S, Croxatto H B, Miranda P, Shaaban M, Sayed E H, Xiao B, Wu S C, Du M, Alvarez F, Brache V, Basnayake S, McCarthy T, Lacarra M, Mishell D R Jr, Koetsawang S, Stern J, Jackanicz T 1997 Contraceptives for lactating women: a comparative trial of a progesterone-releasing vaginal ring and the copper T 380A IUD. Contraception 55:225–232

42. Suherman S K, Affandi B, Korver T 1999 The effects of Implanon on lipid metabolism in comparison with Norplant. Contraception 60:281–287

43. Varma R, Mascarenhas L 2001 Endometrial effects of etonogestrel (Implanon) contraceptive implant. Current Opinions in Obstetrics and Gynecology 13:335–341

44. Vercellini P, De Giorgi O, Mosconi P, Stellato G, Vicentini S, Crosignani P G 2002 Cyproterone acetate versus a continuous monophasic oral contraceptive in the treatment of recurrent pelvic pain after conservative surgery for symptomatic endometriosis. Fertility and Sterility 77:52–61

45. Victor A, Jackanicz T M, Johansson E D 1978 Vaginal progesterone for contraception. Fertility and Sterility 30:631–635

46. Westhoff C 1996 Depot medroxyprogesterone acetate contraception. Metabolic parameters and mood changes. Journal of Reproductive Medicine 41(5 Suppl):401–406

47. Winkler U H, Howie H, Buhler K, Korver T, Geurts T B, Coelingh Bennink H J 1998 A randomized controlled double-blind study of the effects on hemostasis of two progestogen-only pills containing 75 microgram desogestrel or 30 microgram levonorgestrel. Contraception 57:385–392

48. World Health Organization 1983 Multinational comparative clinical trial of long-acting injectable contraceptives: norethisterone enanthate given in two dosage regimens and depot-medroxyprogesterone acetate. Final report. Contraception 28:1–20

7

☆☆☆☆☆☆☆☆☆☆☆☆☆☆☆☆☆☆ | ☆

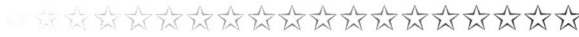

Emergency contraception

James T. McVicker   Anne Webb

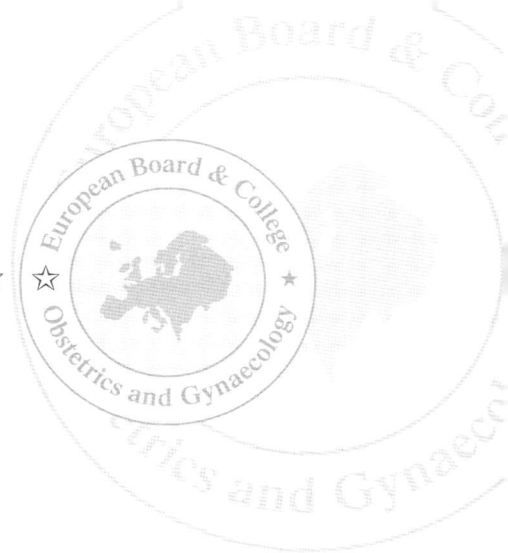

ABSTRACT

When used within the correct time scale modern methods of emergency contraception have been shown to be an effective means of reducing the risk of pregnancy following unprotected sexual intercourse. There are essentially no contraindications to treatment apart from an existing pregnancy. Hormonal methods have an excellent safety record. Major side effects are rare, particularly with newer progestogen-only regimens. Fitting an emergency intrauterine device offers the most effective method and also has the advantage of providing reliable long-term contraception.

Use of emergency contraception could play a major role in reducing the number of unplanned pregnancies worldwide and reduce the significant mortality and morbidity associated with unsafe abortion, yet uptake is low. There is a need to identify barriers to use and develop ways to provide rapid, easy access to emergency contraception for those who need it.

KEYWORDS

Emergency contraception, hormonal, IUD, indications, mechanism, side effects, effectiveness, access, availability

INTRODUCTION

The idea of emergency contraception (EC) or postcoital contraception (PCC) has been in existence since biblical times. Serfaty gives numerous examples.[11] The early Egyptians favoured a concoction of wine, garlic and fennel as a vaginal douche immediately after coitus whereas later civilisations recommended a series of violent exercises for the female partner. It is only since the 1960s that more reliable methods based on contraceptive steroid hormones have been developed. The copper intrauterine device (IUD) has been used for EC since the 1970s. Initial high-dose oestrogen regimens (5 mg ethinylestradiol for five days) were abandoned in favour of a combination of ethinylestradiol and levonorgestrel, developed by Yuzpe and Lancee.[22] Approved by the Committee on Safety of Medicines for use in the United Kingdom (UK) in 1984, this method was the main form of hormonal EC until early this century. In 1998, the *Lancet* published a report[18] from a World Health Organization (WHO) multicentre trial, which confirmed the efficacy of a progestogen-only method, initially developed by Ho and Kwan.[8] With the recent licensing and distribution of a levonorgestrel preparation, this has become the hormonal method of choice in the UK and in other countries where it is available.

INDICATIONS FOR USING EC

The aim of EC is to try to prevent pregnancy after unprotected sexual intercourse (UPSI) has taken place. This need may arise either because intercourse has occurred without using any contraception or because of a potential failure of the client's normal method. Determining the risk of pregnancy in any given situation may be difficult.[13] Where no regular contraception is being used, there is a 30% risk of pregnancy following sexual intercourse on the days before and just after ovulation. The risk at other times in the cycle is considerably less (±3%) but no risk of pregnancy can ever be guaranteed. Much depends on the regularity of the cycle and the client's accurate recall of the dates of her last menses. In the situation of missed pills it may be even more difficult to assess this risk. Even when the risk of pregnancy occurring appears low, it may be better to provide some form of EC rather than not, particularly if the client's anxiety levels are high.

Guidelines from the Faculty of Family Planning and Reproductive Health Care (FFPRHC)[3] give a detailed account of the indications for consideration of the need for EC. These are summarised below:

UNPROTECTED SEX

This usually refers to consensual sexual intercourse where no contraceptive method has been used. It should also include coitus interruptus and any situation where ejaculation has occurred on the external genitalia. It is essential to consider EC use in cases of rape or sexual assault.

POTENTIAL BARRIER METHOD FAILURES

Condom rupture or dislodgement; incorrect insertion of diaphragm; device damaged, dislodged during intercourse or removed too early.

MISSED CONTRACEPTIVE PILLS WHEN ADDITIONAL METHODS NOT USED/FAILED

All pill users should be made aware of what to do in the event of missed pills when they first start to use the method. Up-to-date information on advice for combined oral contraceptives (COC) can be found in *Guidelines on First Prescription of Combined Oral Contraception* from the FFPRHC.[4] Progestogen-only pills (POP) should be taken within three hours of the scheduled time each day. If one or more pills are missed or are taken more than three hours late (more than 12 hours for the newer desogestrel-based POP), the WHO advises that additional barrier contraception is necessary until pills have been taken correctly for two consecutive days (48 hours). EC should be considered if this advice is not followed or if the recommended additional measures fail in the following situations.

Combined pills*
- Two or more pills missed from the first seven in a packet.
- Four or more pills missed mid-packet.

EC is not necessary if two or more pills are missed from the last seven in the packet, provided that the subsequent pill-free interval is omitted.

Progestogen-only pills
- One or more pills taken more than three hours (12 hours for the newer desogestrel-based pills) after usual pill-taking time or missed completely and UPSI has occurred in the two days after this.

DRUG INTERACTIONS REDUCING EFFICACY OF HORMONAL CONTRACEPTIVE METHODS

Short-term use of broad spectrum antibiotics may reduce the efficacy of COCs, therefore clients should be advised to use additional barrier methods during antibiotic use and for seven days afterwards. Broad-spectrum antibiotics do not affect the efficacy of POPs. Liver-enzyme-inducing drugs, e.g. carbamazepine, may affect the efficacy of both COCs and POPs. Clients using liver-enzyme-inducing drugs may require a larger dose of hormonal EC (see Interactions with other drugs, p. 122). EC should be considered in the following situations.

Combined pills
- Failed barrier method or UPSI during short-term antibiotic use or in the seven days after finishing the course.
- Failed barrier method or UPSI during, or in the 28 days after, the use of enzyme-inducing drugs.

---

*The most recent updated information concerning missed combined pills can be obtained from the Clinical Effectiveness Unit of the Faculty of Family Planning and Reproductive Health Care. This may be accessed on the Faculty website at www.ffprhc.org.uk

Progestogen-only pills

- Failed barrier method or UPSI during, or in the 28 days after, the use of enzyme-inducing drugs.

Progestogen-only implants

- Failed barrier method or UPSI during, or in the 28 days after, the use of enzyme-inducing drugs.

LATE INJECTIONS WITH DEPO-MEDROXYPROGESTERONE ACETATE (DMPA)

DMPA is the injection of choice in the UK and is licensed to provide contraceptive cover for up to 89 days. Recent advice from the WHO,[19] supported by the FFPRHC,[3] suggests that contraceptive cover extends up to 14 weeks since the last injection. Therefore EC may need to be considered only if the injection is more than 14 weeks since the last injection and UPSI has taken place.

POTENTIAL IUD FAILURE

Where a routine device has been partially or completely expelled spontaneously or where it is deemed necessary to remove an IUD and sexual intercourse has taken place within the previous five days.

RECENT USE OF POSSIBLE TERATOGENS

Concomitant use of cytotoxic drugs or live vaccines.

METHODS AVAILABLE

As mentioned in the introduction, a number of methods of EC may be considered. Specific licensed products may not be available in all countries. In the absence of such products it is common practice to use combinations of standard oral contraceptive pills to achieve the required dose, acknowledging, of course, that this use is outside the product license.

ETHINYLESTRADIOL

High-dose estrogen regimens were the basis of early studies in the 1960s. Ethinylestradiol 5 mg daily for five days has been shown to be effective[7] if treatment is started within 72 hours of coitus. The main problem with this regimen is a high incidence of nausea and vomiting and prophylactic anti-emetics may be necessary. Concerns have been raised about a higher risk of ectopic pregnancy in the event of failure of the method. Due to the theoretical association between estrogen and venous thromboembolic disorders, it may be considered unsuitable for use in those individuals at increased risk. It is now rarely used in the UK, having been superseded by what are considered safer regimens.

COMBINED ESTROGEN/PROGESTOGEN METHOD

The Yuzpe regimen[22] consists of 100 μg ethinylestradiol and 1000 μg norgestrel (equivalent to 500 μg levonorgestrel) given within 72 hours of coitus and the dose repeated 12 hours later. A licensed product consisting of four tablets, marketed specifically for EC, was formerly available in the UK, Germany, Norway, Sweden, Switzerland, Denmark, Finland, France and Portugal. For many years this was the hormonal method of choice in the UK but it has now been withdrawn from the market as it has been superseded by the progestogen-only method. Many clinicians may prefer to make up their own dose using standard combined pills, e.g. ethinylestradiol 30 μg/levonorgestrel 150 μg × four pills, repeated after 12 hours or ethinylestradiol 50 μg/levonorgestrel 250 μg × two, repeated after 12 hours. The latter version was regularly used in our own clinics over a long period of time and was significantly cheaper than the proprietary product. It also allowed us to provide additional pills to cover the risk of vomiting or interaction with other medication (see later). The 72-hour time limit for initiating treatment is based on Yuzpe's original work. There is some evidence from a recent Population Council study, as yet unpublished, that treatment still has some effect even if started up to five days after coitus.

PROGESTOGEN-ONLY METHOD

A study by Ho and Kwan[8] in 1993 suggested that a regimen of levonorgestrel 750 μg given within 48 hours of coitus and repeated 12 hours later had similar effectiveness to the combined regimen. However, it was not until 1998, following the publication of a much larger WHO multicentre study,[18] that this method gained greater popularity. The standard progestogen-only regimen is now 750 μg of levonorgestrel given within 72 hours of coitus and repeated after 12 hours. A proprietary product consisting of two levonorgestrel 750 μg tablets is now available in the UK, France, Spain, Finland and Hungary. Prior to this product becoming available in the UK, many clinicians made up an equivalent dose using standard progestogen-only pills (POP), e.g. levonorgestrel 30 μg × 25 tablets repeated after 12 hours or norgestrel 75 μg × 20 tablets repeated after 12 hours. Despite the need to take such a large number of tablets, this regimen proved more popular amongst our clients, particularly those who had previously used the Yuzpe method. Associated nausea and vomiting was significantly less. A WHO study[14] published in 2002 suggested that taking both tablets of levonorgestrel 750 μg at the same time, rather than 12 hours apart, may be just as effective in preventing pregnancy. This is now reflected in the summary of product characteristics of the licensed product in the UK.

THE INTRAUTERINE DEVICE

Postcoital insertion of a copper-containing IUD has been shown to be an extremely effective method of EC with a failure rate of less than 0.1%.[12] It may be fitted up to five days after a single episode of intercourse or up to five days after the earliest estimated date of ovulation, calculated on the basis of the woman's shortest menstrual cycle. Therefore, if intercourse has occurred before ovulation, a copper-containing IUD may still be fitted more than five days after intercourse, even if there have been multiple episodes of risk, provided that it is no more than five days after the estimated time of ovulation.

This method has the added advantage of providing immediate ongoing contraception. The device may be removed following the onset of the next menstruation or it may be left in situ if the woman wishes to use it for reliable long-term contraception.

Only a copper-containing IUD should be used. The levonorgestrel-containing intrauterine-system device has not been shown to be effective for EC.

OTHER METHODS STUDIED

Several other oral methods have been studied including danazol and mifepristone.

Danazol

Early studies implied that this antigonadotrophin and progestogen had potential for use as EC. However, a randomised trial using danazol 600 µg, given within 72 hours of unprotected intercourse and repeated after 12 hours, in comparison with the Yuzpe regimen,[15] failed to show any clinical effect. It is not recommended as a method of EC.

Mifepristone

A study[15] using the antiprogestogen mifepristone 600 mg given as a single dose within 72 hours of unprotected intercourse, showed it to be significantly more effective than the Yuzpe regimen. It was associated with a lower incidence of side effects but caused greater delay in the onset of subsequent menstruation. The fact that this dose is the same as that used to act as an abortifacient may make it politically sensitive in some countries. A further WHO study[20] comparing three doses (600 mg, 50 mg and 10 mg) of mifepristone, with treatment initiated up to 120 hours after unprotected intercourse, showed similar efficacy for all three groups. Efficacy was higher in those receiving treatment within three days. The more recent WHO study[14] comparing mifepristone 10 mg with two regimens of levonorgestrel has confirmed these results.

MECHANISMS OF ACTION

Research into in-vitro fertilisation over the last 20 years has shown that the whole process of fertilisation and subsequent successful pregnancy is much more complicated than previously thought. Exactly how the various methods of EC work is still a subject for debate.

HORMONAL METHODS

Several mechanisms have been suggested. The mode of action may depend on when in the cycle treatment occurs. If given in the follicular phase of the cycle, before ovulation occurs, then ovulation may be prevented or delayed. This is thought to be due to interference with the pre-ovulatory peak and luteinising hormone surge. Normal functioning of the corpus luteum may be disturbed, affecting ovum transport and fertilisation. Hormonal effects on the endometrium may make it hostile to sperm penetration and may also inhibit implantation. There is no evidence that hormonal methods interfere with an already established pregnancy.

COPPER IUD

Again a number of possible modes of action have been described. When used as a long-term method of contraception copper-releasing IUDs are known to have an effect on the endometrium, interfering with sperm transport and also interfering with the ability of sperm to fertilise an egg. Copper may have an adverse affect on ovulation and the viability of the egg and cause endometrial changes, which may inhibit implantation. Some or all of these mechanisms may account for the emergency contraceptive action, depending on the stage of the cycle when the device is fitted.

An understanding of how the method works may be of importance to the woman when deciding whether or not to use EC. Those who do not wish to use a post-fertilisation pre-implantation method may choose not to proceed.

EFFECTIVENESS

Most studies of EC methods have reported results in terms of either a failure rate (the proportion of women becoming pregnant despite treatment) or as the ratio of the number of observed pregnancies to the number of expected pregnancies without treatment. Trussell and Ellerton[12] outline the problems of designing suitable trials to assess the efficacy of EC. Participants should have accurate recall of cycle data and coital history. Ensuring low numbers lost to follow-up is important to determine pregnancy rate in the treatment cycle. It should also be remembered that the majority of women using EC at any particular time would not necessarily have become pregnant without treatment.

HORMONAL METHODS

A study[13] reviewing ten trials looking at the efficacy of the Yuzpe regimen showed considerable variation in the estimated effectiveness. However, pooling of the results of these ten trials suggested that using this regimen, within 72 hours of UPSI, could reduce the likelihood of pregnancy by 75%.

A more recent WHO study[18] comparing the efficacy of the levonorgestrel-only method with that of the Yuzpe regimen suggested that the levonorgestrel-only method was more effective (85% vs. 57% of pregnancies prevented), when treatment was started within 72 hours of risk. This study quotes a lower efficacy rate for the Yuzpe regimen compared with other studies and there has been some debate concerning both trial design and the interpretation of the results. Certainly the levonorgestrel method has been shown to be at least as effective as the Yuzpe regimen.

TIMING OF STARTING TREATMENT

This study[18] also confirmed the importance of timing of the first dose of treatment. Both methods were shown to be more effective when treatment started within 24 hours of unprotected intercourse (Table 7.1). These results have implications in terms of service provision, with respect to health-delivery services and deciding from where EC should be available. A further WHO study[14] suggested that the levonorgestrel method may be effective for up to 120 hours of UPSI. Ideally women should be advised to take hormonal EC as soon as possible after any episode of risk.

INTERACTIONS WITH OTHER DRUGS

Drug interactions may occur with hormonal EC in women already using other medications. We have already mentioned that liver-enzyme-inducing drugs can increase metabolism of standard oral contraceptive pills, potentially interfering with efficacy. How significant this may be with EC preparations is not known. Use of an IUD may be a better option in this situation. When hormonal EC is used in this situation, it has been our practice to empirically use a 50% or 100% higher dose given initially and, if tolerated, a similarly high second dose. Alternatively three tablets of levonorgestrel 750 μg may be given as a single dose. Common enzyme-inducing drugs include rifampicin, phenytoin, barbiturates and carbamazepine. It is important to remember that some herbal preparations are enzyme inducers, e.g. St John's Wort.

Broad-spectrum antibiotics may interfere with estrogen absorption and potentially could affect the Yuzpe regimen. This is not a problem with the levonorgestrel regimen.

It should also be remembered that use of hormonal EC does not give protection against pregnancy for the rest of the menstrual cycle. Women must be advised to use a reliable form of contraception or abstain from sexual intercourse until the onset of the next menstruation.

Table 7.1 Percentage of expected pregnancies prevented vs. time interval from coitus to treatment

Coitus to treatment time (hours)	Progestogen-only regimen (%)	Combined (Yuzpe) regimen (%)
24 or less	95	77
25–48	85	36
49–72	58	31

THE IUD

As already stated, using a copper-containing IUD for EC has a failure rate of <0.1%,[12] making it the most effective method. Despite this and the fact that it can be fitted within a longer time from an episode of risk, it is not commonly used outside of specialist contraceptive services in the UK.

CONTRAINDICATIONS TO THE USE OF EC

There are essentially no contraindications to EC[21] other than pregnancy. It is important to carefully assess each request for EC to exclude any possibility of an already existing pregnancy.

CONTRAINDICATIONS SPECIFIC TO HORMONAL METHODS

For years the WHO has stated that there are no medical contraindications to hormonal EC apart from established pregnancy and that is only because the method would obviously not be effective. Earlier versions of the FFPRHC Guidelines expressed concerns about use of the Yuzpe regimen in women with a history of thromboembolic disease or those who presented with an acute episode of focal migraine. These initial concerns were based on extrapolation of knowledge of long-term use of the combined oral contraceptive pill. Although the dose of ethinylestradiol in the Yuzpe method is higher, the duration of treatment is short. Studies[16,17] have failed to show any adverse effect on clotting factors associated with short duration of treatment and this has been borne out by clinical practice. Some individuals may have a higher risk of thromboembolic disease, e.g. because of abnormal clotting factors, and this could be considered a relative rather than absolute contraindication. In this situation the levonorgestrel-only regimen or an IUD may be the preferred option.

A similar approach may be considered in women with a history of migraine associated with transient neurological symptoms, crescendo migraine or on treatment with ergotamine or who has a migraine at time of presentation.

Concerns about a possible increased risk of ectopic pregnancy occurring may stem from use of the older ethinylestradiol 5 mg for five days regimen,[7] which provided a much higher dose of estrogen. This has not been seen in clinical practice over many years. Those individuals already at higher risk of ectopic pregnancy, i.e. with a past history of ectopic pregnancy or known to have significant tubal damage, should be warned that in the event of failure of the method, an ectopic pregnancy should be excluded.

Similarly, concerns about use of estrogen and teratogenesis seem unfounded. In the event of pregnancy occurring despite treatment within 72 hours, there is evidence that the pre-implantation embryo is resistant to teratogenesis.[1] Where treatment may be given inadvertently in early pregnancy a WHO review[21] suggests that any teratogenic risk would be very small if present at all. Obviously, as stated above, if pregnancy was already thought likely, then EC would be avoided.

Since, as already stated, there is no evidence that either regimen has any adverse effect on a continuing pregnancy in the event of failure, such a failure would not, in itself, be an indication for termination of pregnancy.

There are similarly no contraindications to the use of the progestogen-only method, apart from an established pregnancy. The latter reflects its lack of effect on an established pregnancy rather than concerns about teratogenicity.

If using proprietary hormonal products marketed specifically for EC, clinicians should refer to the summary of product characteristics in the manufacturer's guidelines.

CONTRAINDICATIONS SPECIFIC TO THE COPPER-CONTAINING IUD

WHO eligibility criteria[21] list only pre-existing pregnancy as an absolute contraindication to use of this method. Current sexually transmitted infection (STI) or a high risk of STI is listed as Class 3, where theoretical or proven risks outweigh any advantage.

Risk of STI

Women requesting EC often forget the fact that an episode of UPSI may have put them at risk of STI, concentrating instead on the risk of pregnancy. This is particularly important if considering using a postcoital IUD as it may increase the risk of pelvic inflammatory disease (PID). The fact that an IUD may be fitted up to five days after exposure to risk may allow time for an individual to attend a specialist genitourinary medicine (GUM) service for assessment and initiation of treatment if necessary, prior to fitting within the required time scale. This also allows for proper contact tracing to be arranged. Other alternatives are:

- Take relevant swabs, e.g. for chlamydia or other STIs known to be prevalent locally, immediately prior to fitting the device and arrange follow-up as soon as results are available and deal with results as necessary.
- Once swabs have been taken and the device fitted, give prophylactic antibiotics either as a one-off dose or longer course.

Use of prophylactic antibiotics alone, without taking swabs, does not allow for contact tracing. Decision about which approach to take should be based on knowledge of the local prevalence of common STIs and the availability of GUM services.

Ability to fit an IUD

All types of copper-containing IUDs have been used for EC although most are not licensed for this purpose. Clinicians fitting IUDs should have had proper training in the techniques involved and should be able to deal with complications that may arise. Perforation of the uterus is rare in experienced hands but cervical shock, as a result of dilating the cervix, is not uncommon. It is our practice always to have two experienced members of clinical staff present for all IUD fittings with the necessary resuscitation drugs and equipment close to hand.

Nulliparity is not a contraindication to use, although less-experienced inserters may prefer to refer on for such procedures. Fitting a device in women who have had previous surgery to the cervix, e.g. loop excision or knife cone biopsy, may be more difficult and require some degree of cervical dilatation under local anaesthetic. This may be better done in more experienced hands.

SIDE EFFECTS

NAUSEA AND VOMITING

These are common side effects reported with the combined regimen. However, a WHO study[18] showed a significant reduction of both with the progestogen-only regimen (Table 7.2). Prophylactic use of an anti-emetic may be considered, particularly if there is a history of severe nausea and vomiting with previous use. Domperidone 10 mg orally would be the drug of choice as it does not readily cross the blood–brain barrier and thus is less likely to cause extra-pyramidal side effects. Vomiting within two hours of taking either dose of both hormonal methods may necessitate a repeat course of treatment or consideration of the use of an emergency IUD.

Table 7.2 Comparison of side-effect profiles

Side effects	Progestogen-only regimen (%)	Combined regimen (%)
Nausea	23.0	50.5
Vomiting	5.6	18.8

BLEEDING PATTERN

Many women and some clinicians are under the impression that using hormonal EC will induce menstrual bleeding within the next one or two days. Whilst some spotting is not unusual, this is unlikely to be the onset of menstruation. A variety of disturbances to timing of onset of the next menstruation have been described[15] depending on the hormonal method used. A study comparing the efficacy of the Yuzpe regimen with that of the levonorgestrel-only regimen[18] found that, for the majority (57%), menses started within three days of the expected date. Of the rest, 15% started early, 15% were up to seven days late and the remaining 13% were more than seven days late.

REPEATED USE OF EC

Repeated requests for EC usually apply to hormonal methods. Table 7.3 shows the pattern of repeat attenders at a city-centre clinic in Liverpool over a ten-month period. There is no evidence that repeated use causes any harm but it is a major indication that the individual needs to sort out reliable long-term contraception. Repeated use may upset the menstrual cycle, making assessment

Table 7.3 Pattern of repeat attendances for EC at city centre clinic in Liverpool, UK

1 April 2000 to 28 February 2001		Individuals attending more than once for hormonal EC	
Clients attending for EC		Two times	421
Hormonal	3745	Three times	103
IUD	400	Four times	22
Total	4145	Five times	10
		Six times	1
		Seven times	3
		Ten times	1

of further risks of pregnancy more difficult. Statistically, the risk of failure may increase with repeated use.

Repeated use within the same cycle may also be an option, although this is not recommended in the summary of product characteristics of proprietary products. Each request should be carefully considered, assessing the potential risks of giving a small dose of hormones with no known teratogenic potential to a woman who may already be pregnant against the benefits of preventing an unplanned pregnancy.

Discussing ongoing contraception is an important part of managing a request for EC and may depend on what emergency method has been chosen and what was being used immediately prior to the episode of risk. It is important to remember that hormonal EC itself does not provide any ongoing contraception.

DEALING WITH A REQUEST FOR EC

Making a request for EC is often embarrassing for women. Having to admit to what may be perceived as some sort of failure and to discuss intimate details of recent sexual behaviour may actually deter many women from seeking help. The clinician's approach should be sympathetic, supportive and non-judgemental from the start. Ultimately, the choice of whether or not to use EC, and if so, which method to use, should rest with the woman. This must be an informed choice. The clinician must gather all the relevant information to assess the situation and then discuss it fully with the woman so that she may make her own decision.

WHAT THE CLINICIAN NEEDS TO KNOW

The clinician needs to determine the following:

- The first day of the last menstrual period.
- Usual length of menstrual cycle.
- When the first episode of UPSI occurred.
- Any aspects of the woman's medical history that may influence choice of EC method.

Knowledge of the normal cycle will help to estimate the time of possible ovulation and give some indication of the risk of pregnancy. However, as already pointed out (Indications for using EC, p. 116), a lack of risk can never be guaranteed. There may be some occasions when, after considering the facts, EC is not medically necessary, e.g. one or two missed oral contraceptive pills mid-packet. A detailed explanation and advice may negate the need for treatment. However, regardless of how low the estimated risk is, many women may remain anxious and it is reasonable to provide treatment. In such instances, the levonorgestrel-only method could be a good choice.

Where UPSI has occurred more than 72 hours before presentation an emergency IUD will provide a more effective option. Women in this situation may not want to have an IUD fitted, despite being aware of its better efficacy. It may still be worth considering a hormonal method in this situation. Most studies to date have only looked at efficacy when used within 72 hours of risk. There is some recent evidence from a Population Council Study of the Yuzpe regimen suggesting benefit when used up to five days after risk. Similarly, there is evidence[14] that the levonorgestrel method may have some benefit up to five days.

As already stated, there are essentially no contraindications to EC other than an established pregnancy. If the woman is uncertain of the date of onset of her last menstruation or the history is vague, then it may be worth checking a urinary human chorionic gonadotropin (hCG) level. Vaginal examination to exclude pregnancy is rarely justified in this situation. It can not exclude early pregnancy and concern about the need for such examinations may deter individuals from seeking help, especially among younger women.

An accurate medical history should help to identify those women with any significant problems (see Contraindications to the use of EC, p. 124) that might influence the choice of method.

WHAT THE WOMAN NEEDS TO KNOW

The woman needs all the relevant information to help her to make an informed choice. It is an opportunity to allay her concerns and to dispel rumours and myths concerning EC. Having decided that there is a need for EC it is important to discuss the various methods available giving an honest appraisal of the potential risks and benefits of each.

Possible mode of action should be explained in simple terms as concerns about EC being an abortifacient may make it unacceptable to some people.

Hormonal EC

If a hormonal method is chosen it is important to explain about the possible side effects and what might happen to the woman's menstrual pattern. Individuals cope much better with situations when they know what to expect, and are aware of what is normal and what is not. When the pills should be taken and what to do in the event of vomiting within two hours of taking pills should be explained.

The fact that hormonal EC does not provide ongoing contraception should be stressed and more long-term options should also be discussed.

In our service we do not routinely review all those attending for EC. Women are advised to return if they have not had a normal menstrual period within the next three weeks so that pregnancy can be excluded.

Copper IUD

If a copper IUD is the chosen method then it is essential to explain the fitting procedure in detail. The woman must know what to expect and be allowed to be in control of the situation so that she can stop the procedure at any time if she changes her mind. Taking a little time to establish a trusting relationship with the woman will often make the procedure much easier for both her and the clinician. If the device is being used only for EC arrangements should be made for removal after the onset of the next menses. If the device is to be used also as a long-term method of contraception then arrangements for review may be made, in keeping with your normal practice after IUD fitting.

Failure of EC

Women should be advised to return for further assessment if they have not had a normal menstrual period within three weeks of using EC, whatever the method. In this case it is important to estimate urinary hCG levels to exclude the possibility of pregnancy. Whether or not a termination of pregnancy would be considered would depend on the woman's wishes and local laws concerning abortion. The fact that EC had been used is not a relevant factor in making that decision.

Other issues

A consultation for EC must deal adequately with the presenting problem. It also provides an opportunity to consider other issues.

It is important to discuss, at least briefly, the need for reliable on-going and long-term contraception. It may not always be appropriate to go into details at the time but further appointments can be arranged once the initial panic has been resolved. Where the request for EC has been due to missed pills, a woman should be advised to throw away the missed pills and continue with the rest of the packet. She should abstain from intercourse or use condoms until seven consecutive COC pills or two consecutive POPs have been taken to ensure contraceptive cover. A woman wishing to start hormonal contraception should usually be advised to wait until the first day of the next menstruation but, depending on the circumstances, it may be possible to start such methods at the same time as taking EC. Each situation should be assessed individually.

Whilst individuals requesting EC are concerned about the risk of pregnancy few ever consider that they may also be at risk of having been exposed to an STI. Introducing such an idea into what may be an already highly charged situation may seem difficult but it can be done in a non-threatening way. It is essential to consider the possibility if contemplating the use of an IUD (see Risk of STI, p. 124) but should be discussed in all consultations. Appropriate referral for assessment can be arranged if necessary depending on local facilities.

BARRIERS TO USE OF EC

A recent editorial[10] in the *European Journal of Contraception and Reproductive Health Care* suggests that, despite the fact that EC has been in existence in many countries for many years, it is not commonly used. Why should this be?

AWARENESS OF METHOD

A lack of general public awareness of, or knowledge about, the existence of EC has been suggested as a major problem in the past. There is good evidence that this is changing in the UK. A nationwide survey of women aged 15–50 years[2] showed that 91% were aware of the existence of hormonal EC and 48% had heard of the emergency IUD. Our own experience in Liverpool confirms this increasing awareness. In 1999, a request for EC was the main reason given by 20% of women attending our city-centre clinic. A significant increase in the use of EC within our service over recent years is shown in Fig 7.1. Further confirmation of increasing awareness comes from a study[6] of women attending for termination of pregnancy. However this study suggested that, despite increasing awareness, many women still did not use EC. Some were possibly not aware of their risk of pregnancy, suggesting a need to improve overall sex education. Many women, although aware of the risk of pregnancy, still did not use EC possibly due to concerns about the potential risks involved and the difficulties of obtaining it.

There is still a need to increase awareness. Clinicians involved in providing contraceptive services should discuss EC as part of all routine consultations. It should be an essential part of every pill teach and is particularly important to

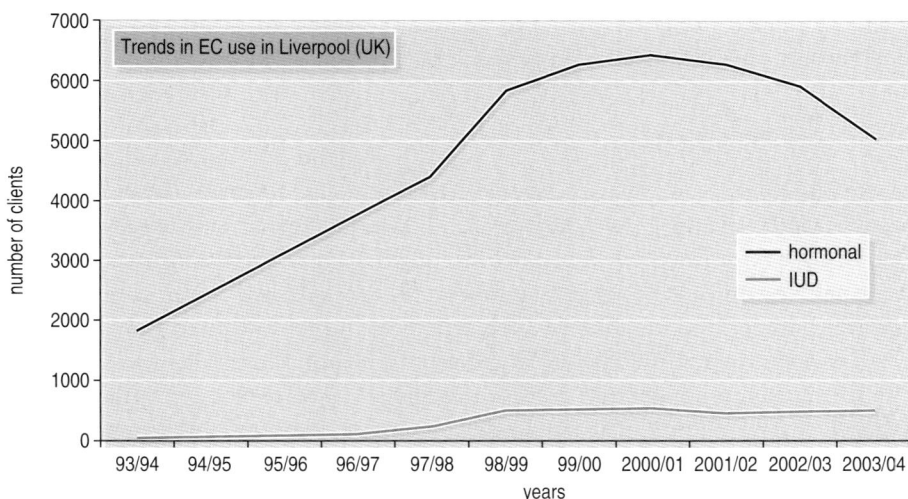

Fig 7.1 Trends in EC use in Abacus Clinics in Liverpool, UK, over the last 10 years.

those individuals for whom condoms are the only method of contraception. It is important to dispel myths about the risks involved and give clear information about how and when EC should be used.

Sex education in schools varies considerably from one country to the next and may vary within any one country. Young people are a particular target group and involving schools and teachers would be a major benefit. Obviously there may be political and religious opposition but supporting teachers in this situation by providing information is a way forward.

Using the media is another potential way of improving information. People often put more trust in what they see in their favourite television programme or magazine rather than in what they are told by their doctor. Including sexual health issues as part of the story line in several UK television 'soap operas' recently has been shown to have a beneficial effect on public opinion. It is essential, however, to ensure that the information given by the media is actually correct.

Improving awareness and accurate knowledge among clinicians and other health professionals is also important. Those professionals not familiar with current knowledge may do more harm than good. Training should not only deal with knowledge of methods but should also include aspects on communication skills and how to deal with consultations.

ATTITUDES

Negative attitudes in both the clinician and the potential user will have an impact on the uptake of EC. In many cultures talking about sex is seen as difficult. For women, requesting EC will be an embarrassing experience made worse by concerns about the possibly judgmental attitudes of clinicians. Fear of having to discuss intimate details, fear of being considered irresponsible or in some way immoral, may all deter use. Some clinicians may have ethical concerns about EC and impose these on others.

There is an overwhelming need to change the image of EC. It should be promoted as a positive, responsible approach to a potential problem.

ACCESS/AVAILABILITY

Having the necessary information is one thing, being able to access services may be something else. In the UK everyone should be registered with a general practitioner (GP) who provides a 24-hour service therefore, in theory, obtaining EC should be easy. In practice this may not be the case. Access to GP surgeries can be limited, appointments take time to arrange and many women may be reluctant to explain the nature of their emergency to receptionists. Many women, particularly those in younger age groups, may have concerns about confidentiality. Family planning clinics may be limited geographically and by clinic opening times. Hospital accident and emergency departments are open 24 hours a day but waiting times may be long and staff perceptions of the level of emergency may differ from those seeking EC.

Improving availability

Perhaps the best way of improving availability of EC is to demedicalise it. Hormonal EC, particularly the levonorgestrel method, has been shown to be safe and virtually free from side effects. Women should not necessarily need to see a doctor to obtain it.

Since 1994, appropriately trained nurses in our service have been issuing hormonal EC to women according to a set protocol. An initial review of the service after several years[9] showed a significant fall in the proportion of women being referred on to see a doctor. The protocol has been further developed to allow nurses to issue ongoing long-term contraception as well. The system works exceptionally well, allowing us to cope with ever-increasing numbers of clients and still maintain a quality service. It allows better use of the individual skills of nurses and doctors and improves overall 'job satisfaction'.

More recently in the UK the licensing of a levonorgestrel-only product, specifically manufactured for EC, has been changed from a prescription only medicine to a pharmacist medicine. A woman may now purchase hormonal EC over the counter at a pharmacy. Initial objections from some clinicians were based more on moral issues or concerns about losing control of prescribing. Some seemed to think that it would be abused in some way, e.g. used too often or used to induce abortion. Once again this was more a reflection of individuals' attitudes or perceptions of women who might use EC rather than based on any evidence. As a result of collaboration between representative groups guidelines for pharmacists have been drawn up to ensure simple but safe provision but avoiding unnecessary interrogation. Pharmacists should also be able to supply relevant information about possible need for follow-up and local contraception services. Whereas, in the UK, all contraceptive provision from GPs and community-based contraceptive services is free, there is a charge for the pharmacy product. It has been suggested that those most in need may not be able to afford to buy it. Despite this, within six months of the launch of the pharmacy product, although overall sales of hormonal EC have only increased very slightly, the pharmacy product accounts for 25% of all sales. Following several pilot studies, a number of pharmacies in different parts of the UK are now able to provide hormonal EC to women of all ages free of charge.

Some studies[5] have looked at the feasibility of providing women with a supply of hormonal EC to keep at home in case of need. Contrary to the concerns of some health professionals there was no evidence that it was used 'improperly'.

We must continue to explore all avenues to provide rapid easy access to EC.

Useful Internet websites
www.ffprhc.org.uk
Faculty of Family Planning and Reproductive Health Care of the Royal College of Obstetricians and Gynaecologists. Click on publications for access to a wide range of guidelines on all aspects of contraception.

www.who.int

WHO website. Click on site index and then on reproductive health, enter 'medical eligibility criteria' and search, review the table of contents.

References

1. Austin C R 1973 Embryo transfer and sensitivity to teratogenesis. Nature 244:333–334
2. Dawe F, Meltzer H 2001 Contraception and sexual health 1999: a report on research for the Department of Health using the ONS Omnibus Survey. Office for National Statistics, London
3. FFPRHC Guidance April 2003 updated June 2003 Emergency contraception. Journal of Family Planning and Reproductive Health Care 29(2)
4. FFPRHC Guidance October 2003 First prescription of combined oral contraception. Journal of Family Planning and Reproductive Health Care 29(4)
5. Glasier A, Baird D 1998 The effects of self-administering emergency contraception. New England Journal of Medicine 339:1–4
6. Gordon A, Owen P 1999 Emergency contraception: change in knowledge of women attending for termination of pregnancy from 1984 1996. The British Journal of Family Planning 24:121–122
7. Haspels A A 1976 Interception: post-coital estrogens in 3016 women. Contraception 14:375–381
8. Ho P C, Kwan M S 1993 A prospective randomised comparison of levonorgestrel with the Yuzpe regimen in post-coital contraception. Human Reproduction 8:389–392
9. Jarvis R R, Webb A, Kishen M 1996 Provision of emergency contraception by nurse: a way forward to increased access. European Journal of Contraception and Reproductive Health Care 1:257–262
10. Lech M M, Bonati G 2001 Editorial: the need for more active promotion of emergency contraception. European Journal of Contraception and Reproductive Health Care 6:65–70
11. Serfaty D 1995 Post-coital contraception: historical background from ancient Egypt to the 1960s. Fertility Control Reviews 4(2):25–28
12. Trussell J, Ellerton C 1995 Efficacy of emergency contraception. Fertility Control Reviews 4(2):9–10
13. Trussell J., Stewart F 1992 The effectiveness of post-coital hormonal contraception. Family Planning Perspectives 2:262–264
14. Von Hertzen H, Piaggio G, Ding J et al 2002 Low-dose mifepristone and two regimens of levonorgestrel for emergency contraception: a WHO multicentre randomised controlled trial. Lancet 360:1803–1810
15. Webb A M C, Russel J, Elstein M 1992 Comparison of Yuzpe regime, danazol and mifepristone (RU486) in oral post-coital contraception. British Medical Journal 305:927–931
16. Webb A, Taberner D 1993 Clotting factors after emergency contraception. Advances in Contraception 9:75–82
17. Weenink G H, Ten Cate J W, Kahle L H 1983 "Morning after pill" and antithrombin III. Acta Obstetricia et Gynecologica Scandinavica 62:359–363
18. World Health Organization Task Force on Postovulatory Methods of Fertility Regulation 1998 Randomised controlled trial of levonorgestrel versus the Yuzpe regimen of combined oral contraceptives for emergency contraception. Lancet 352:428–433
19. World Health Organization 2002 Selected practice recommendations for contraceptive use. WHO, Geneva
20. World Health Organization 1996 Special programme of research, development and research training in human reproduction. Annual technical report. WHO, Geneva
21. World Health Organization 2002 Improving access to quality care in family planning: medical eligibility criteria for initiating and continuing use of contraceptive methods. WHO, Geneva
22. Yuzpe A A, Lancee W J 1977 Ethinylestradiol and dl-norgestrel as a post-coital contraceptive. Fertility and Sterility 28:932–936

8

☆☆☆☆☆☆☆☆☆☆☆☆☆☆☆☆ ☆

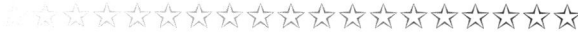

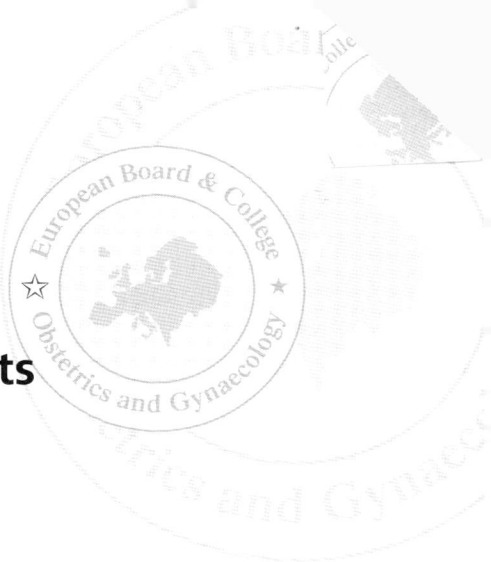

Contraception in adolescents

George Creatsas   Efthimios Deligeoroglou

ABSTRACT

Adolescence is, without doubt, a landmark in every woman's life. The transition from childhood to reproductive age may give rise to serious health-related problems of that age, such as unintended pregnancies and the acquisition of sexually transmitted diseases (STDs), including human immunodeficiency virus (HIV). Adolescents are susceptible to unintended pregnancies, which often force them into unwanted marriage or limit their opportunities for further education or employment while predisposing them to long-term welfare dependence.

Adolescent contraception continues to be a complex and perplexing issue for families, health-care professionals, educators, government officials, and youths themselves. Widespread efforts are made to increase contraceptive use, especially the condom, to prevent both pregnancy and STDs among sexually active teenagers. To be most effective, sex-education programmes should be developed through a process of collaboration between the community, parental organisations, schools, the media and governmental institutions. The organisation of family planning centres for adolescents is undoubtedly necessary and must become a government priority.

KEYWORDS

Adolescence, family planning, contraception

INTRODUCTION

Adolescence is, without doubt, a landmark in every woman's life. The transition from childhood to reproductive age is signalled by a number of important events, such as menarche, acceleration of body development with the appearance of a woman's body characteristics (secondary sexual characteristics). The exploration of sexuality in combination with the lack of knowledge, experience and counselling, may give origin to serious health-related problems of that age, such as unintended pregnancies and the acquisition of sexually transmitted diseases (STDs), including human immunodeficiency virus (HIV). Current rates of sexual activity, pregnancy, and STDs among adolescents remain a public-health concern. Abstaining from intercourse or postponing future sexual relationships is the safest way to prevent STDs and unwanted pregnancy. The age at which first sexual intercourse starts has recently decreased. On the other hand, the percentage of American adolescents who are sexually active has increased significantly in recent years.[17] It is reported that 56% of girls and 73% of boys have had sexual intercourse before the age of 18.[1]

Each year, 75 million unwanted pregnancies occur worldwide. This is mainly due to the non-use of contraception. In addition to that the method used often fails, in at least 8 million cases per year. An estimated 350 million couples around the world lack information about contraceptives; 120–150 million married women who want to limit future pregnancies are not using a contraceptive method; and 12–15 million unmarried women lack the means to do so. Every day 55 000 unsafe abortions take place (95% of them in developing countries). Unsafe abortions are the cause of 200 deaths daily and an unreported number of disabilities. Adolescents are susceptible to unintended pregnancies that often force them into unwanted marriage or limit their opportunities for further education or employment while predisposing them to long-term welfare dependence. Adolescents are frequently uninformed, or misinformed, about sexuality and the risks associated with early and unprotected sexual activity. In developed countries 7.5–10% of adolescent women get pregnant (27% worldwide).[25] Approximately 51% of adolescent pregnancies result in a live birth, 35% of them end with an abortion with several complications, while 14% end in miscarriage or stillbirth.[1,34] Fifty-two percent of adolescents use non-effective contraception.[2] Despite the general reduction of births in the USA, the frequency of pregnancy increases between 14 and 17 years of age. Approximately 31% of adolescents used no contraceptive method at first intercourse, mostly those who had just met their sexual partner.[23]

In Sweden the abortion rate among teenagers has increased by 25% over the past five years. Teenage abortion rates have gone up from 17 per 1000 in 1995 to 22.5 per 1000 in 2001. Genital chlamydial infections have increased from 14 000 cases in 1994 to 22 263 cases in 2001, 60% of these infections occurring among young people, basically among teenagers.[14]

Adolescent contraception continues to be a complex and perplexing issue for families, health-care professionals, educators, government officials, and youths themselves. Widespread efforts are made to increase contraceptive use, especially the condom, to prevent both pregnancy and STDs among sexually active teenagers. Recent studies have found that allowing access to sexual knowledge or birth control in school-based clinics did not affect rates of sexual activity or intercourse at a younger age but did increase use of condoms.[28]

In another study, it was reported that most parents believed that sex education should include information on birth-control methods, including condoms. The information should be provided by the family, supplemented by schools, before students reach the seventh grade. In addition, receiving a regular news-letter regarding teen sexual issues could be of great help to parents in communi-cation with their children.[21] To be most effective, sex-education programmes should be developed through a process of collaboration between the community, parental organisations, schools, the media and governmental institutions.

ADOLESCENT SEXUALITY AND THE MASS MEDIA

Currently, the average American child or adolescent spends 17–21 hours per week viewing television, excluding time spent on watching movies, listening to music or watching music videos, playing video games, or surfing the Internet for recreational purposes.[26] On average, children between 9 and 17 years of age use the Internet four days per week and spend almost two hours on line each time.[27] By the time adolescents graduate from high school, they will have spent 15 000 hours watching television, compared with 12 000 hours spent in the classroom.[32]

American media, both programming and advertising, are highly sexualised in their content. In fact, the average young viewer is exposed to 14 000 sexual refer-ences each year. Only 165 of these deal with responsible sexual behaviour or accu-rate information on birth control matters, abstinence, or the risks of pregnancy and STDs.[2,9] Although early sexual activity may be caused by a variety of factors the media are believed to play a significant role. The media represent the easiest method to influence young people concerning their sexual attitudes and behaviors.[6] There are numerous studies that illustrate television's powerful influence on ado-lescents' sexual attitudes, values, and beliefs.[4] It is suggested that the media should provide messages that support and encourage the delay of first coitus and also pres-ent information on the use of methods to avoid unintended pregnancies and STDs.

THE MALE CONDOM

More than 333 million new cases of the four most curable STDs (gonorrhoea, chlamydia, trichomoniasis, and syphilis) occur annually, mostly in the developing world. Combined oral contraceptives (COCs) should be consistently used in com-bination with the condom as a method of providing complete protection against unwanted pregnancy as well as STDs. Unfortunately, adolescents' dual use of con-doms and hormonal contraceptives is very low.[24] Although the incidence rate of pelvic inflammatory disease (PID) shows over 50% decrease in pill users, the inci-dence of chlamydial and mycoplasmal cervical infections is slightly increased. Unfortunately, the pill offers no protection against viral infections, such as HIV. It is estimated that in the USA approximately 3 million adolescents acquire an STD each year including both bacterial (e.g. gonorrhoea, chlamydia) and viral infections (e.g. herpes, HIV). The rate of STDs among adolescents is increasing. It is reported that 21% of American adolescents have had more than four sexual partners.[20]

Most condoms are made of latex. Polyurethane condoms have recently become available for use. Natural condoms (made of lamb intestine) may be permeable to microorganisms. Spermicides, especially nonoxynol-9, have been recommended as a mean of improving the efficacy of condom use.[18] In favour of this dual use were findings that spermicides not only killed or inactivated sperm but also a great number of other frequently isolated pathogens, but no studies ever proved the effectiveness of spermicides on STD or HIV transmission. Furthermore, spermicides have been implicated as a cause vaginal irritation in some studies.[33]

Despite recent trends towards increased use by adolescents, consistent condom use is reported by less than half of all sexually active adolescents.[29] The most important errors that lead to clinical failure are breakage, slippage, and failure to use throughout intercourse. Breakage and slippage rates of the male condom have each been estimated to be less than 2%, although rates vary among the various studies and according to the user's experience.[30] Condom failure is about ten-times higher among teenagers than adults.[5] It means that condoms cannot be 100% effective, with a theoretical annual failure rate around 2%. Actual failure rates range from 5 to 20%.[18] Goldman et al[16] reported first-year failure rates as low as 2–4% in adolescents. In real-life use, condoms, especially if used consistently and correctly, can be expected to decrease the rates of unintended pregnancy and STD and HIV acquisition among those who are sexually active, including adolescents. The literature findings show that condom use appears to decrease, but does not fully eliminate, the rate of transmission of most STDs. The correct and consistent use of reliable contraception and condoms is a responsibility of both male and female adolescents. In the interest of public health, restrictions and barriers should be removed and schools should be considered as appropriate sites for the availability of condoms.

COMBINED ORAL CONTRACEPTIVES (COCS)

It is widely known that the 'pill' guarantees the highest contraceptive protection. This is the reason that it is a popular contraceptive method around the world. Over 150 000 000 women users are under 30 years old. In some European countries it is used by 50% of women and is considered an appropriate contraceptive method for adolescents. Hormonal contraception is an important issue for the young woman's life. Between 1950, when Gregory Pincus started research on the pill, and the present day the pharmaceutical industry has succeeded in creating contraceptive pills containing low concentrations of estrogens and progestogens, with practically no side effects, thus overcoming issues such as bone growth arrest or weight gain. In addition to protection against an unwanted pregnancy other advantages of the pill's use during adolescence are: the decrease of menorrhagia[11] (blood loss during menses, which is very important when anaemia coexists); reduction of benign breast disease; lowering the severity of endometriosis; suppression of ovarian functional cysts; lowering the severity of PID; decreases in ovarian and endometrial cancer;[13] and reduction of the incidence of ectopic pregnancy. Other important positive effects of hormonal contraception are the relief of dysmenorrhoea,[12] the regulation of menstruation, and the improvement of acne and polycystic ovary syndrome. Furthermore, the pill may postpone menstruation over defined periods of time, such as school exams or during holidays, when bleeding or dysmenorrhoea can create problems. Taking the pill at about the same time every day (every morning just after awakening or every night before going to bed) is recommended in order to create a habit and increase compliance. When pills are properly used, the maximum contraceptive protection is obtained. The COCs' undesired side-effects depend on the dosage of estrogen or the quality of progestogen. These can be: vaginal bleeding (found in pills with low estrogen dose); depression in young girls, when other psychological problems coexist; galactorrhoea or amenorrhoea (in less than 1% of users) after the interruption of the COCs use.

Hormonal contraception should not be prescribed in the following cases: cardiovascular problems; venous thrombosis;[8] liver disease; focal migraine; depression; excessive obesity; and undiagnosed breast mass. Clinical tests concerning metabolism and lipid profiles are rarely necessary during adolescence. In some cases, blood coagulating factors and the liver's function tests are occasionally needed. Incorrect perception that hormonal contraceptive methods are dangerous may originate from breast and pelvic examination during the first consultation, which causes psychological problems. The only areas that truly need to be examined are the medical history and the measurement of blood pressure. For most women no further evaluation is necessary.[31] In comparison with older women, a higher rate of failure is noted during adolescence due to higher frequency of sexual relationships, ideal fertility conditions and, most of all, due to lower compliance to the method and its abandonment or inappropriate use. An explanation for this may be lack of experience and the young girl's immaturity.

DEPO-MEDROXYPROGESTERONE ACETATE (DMPA)

Since its introduction, DMPA, of all the highly effective methods of reversible contraception, offers the longest contraceptive activity. It only requires a single injection every 13 weeks and can be reversed simply by discontinuing injections. DMPA is given in a standard dose of 150 mg intramuscularly every three months and yields a rate of 0–5.2 pregnancies per 1000 woman years.[5] DMPA suppresses the preovulatory surge of luteinising hormone and follicle-stimulating hormone and thereby inhibits ovulation. It is the most suitable method of pregnancy prevention for many women, such as adolescent and adult women who have experienced contraceptive failures or dissatisfaction with other methods.

Despite its excellent safety and efficacy profile, the method has failed to achieve its potential for widespread use, as a result of negative publicity and litigation concerning its side effects. Only time will tell if these concerns have a scientific base. Pre-insertion counselling seems to play an important role in satisfaction and side-effect tolerance.

EMERGENCY CONTRACEPTION

A few years ago, in cases where there was a need for emergency contraception, such as rape or preservative rupture, a high dose of estrogens was in common use but was associated with a high frequency of nausea and vomiting. The Yuzpe regimen is effective and much better tolerated. Danazol, on the other hand, is not so highly effective. Mifepristone has an adverse-effect profile similar to that of the Yuzpe regimen. Furthermore, there is no experience of the use of mifepristone (RU486).[5] During recent years, the efficacy of the progestogen-only pill 'levonorgestrel' as an emergency contraceptive method has been proposed. Levonorgestrel has better results with fewer side effects than previous methods of emergency contraception. A 0.75 mg levonorgestrel pill taken as soon as possible after the insecure intercourse and a second one, taken 12 hours later, is efficient. The efficacy depends on the time span between coitus and pill administration (95% for the first 24 hours, 85% if taken 24–48 hours later, 58% between 48–72 hours later, and nearly no efficacy if more than 72 hours have passed). Awareness of emergency contraception is high among school-age students but knowledge of specific details, such as the recommended time window of effectiveness, is poor. Appropriate use of emergency contraception could prevent up to 75% of unplanned pregnancies.[15,35]

However, lack of knowledge of the method is responsible for the failure of the method. Debate as to whether emergency contraception should be available to teens without a prescription is of great interest. Sexually active women, especially in their teens, seeking emergency hormonal contraception are finding that special family-planning units for adolescents, either in or attached to community hospitals, offer convenience and confidentiality.[19] On the other hand, emergency contraception should not be considered as an alternative regular contraceptive method. The clinician should ensure that the woman uses an effective contraceptive thereafter.

FEMALE CONDOM

The female condom is a new contraceptive method, made of polyurethane, which can be used as an alternative protection by those reporting latex allergy. The method is not popular during adolescence. The device promotes healthy behaviours and increases sexual self-confidence and autonomy. Unfortunately, the disposition of regulatory agencies and the attitudes of health-care providers have reduced access to these methods.

VAGINAL SPONGE

The contraceptive vaginal sponge was developed as an alternative to other barrier methods. It is made of polyurethane and releases 125 mg of the spermicide nonoxynol-9 over 24 hours of use. It can be used for more than one intercourse within 24 hours without changing or adding spermicide and does not require a prescription or fitting by a health-care provider. Other advantages of this method are the control by the woman rather than her partner, the lack of side effects, has antibacterial and antiviral properties, including protection from the HIV,[5] as well as fewer medical contraindications. Unfortunately, the sponge is less effective in preventing pregnancy.[7] Similarly, high discontinuation rates and few allergic-type reactions have been reported.[22]

IMPLANTS AND PATCHES

Implants carrying progestins are made of two types of polymers. Immediately after insertion, they begin to release the progestin in a consistent way. Their effective life varies from 6 to 84 months but the pharmaceutical industry is experimenting on extending this recommended maximum duration of use.[10] This long-term high contraceptive protection makes implants a suitable alternative method for many women.

The transdermal contraceptive patch delivers ethinylestradiol and norelgestromin over seven days, which results in a similar efficacy to that achieved with COCs. Excessive body weight is associated with lower efficacy. The cycle control and side-effect profile is similar to oral contraceptives. A major advantage of this method compared with other methods, even to oral contraceptives, is that it offers nearly 90% perfect compliance to the dosing schedule across all ages. Attachment of the patch is not affected by warm humid climates, vigorous exercise or exposure to saunas or water baths.

MALE HORMONAL CONTRACEPTION

Options for male hormonal fertility control could improve family planning. New methods will come into practise probably within the next few years. Spermatogenesis is dependent on the pituitary gonadotropins. Administration of a high dose of testosterone suppresses gonadotropins and spermatogenesis with an efficacy comparable to female oral contraceptives, resulting in reversible azoospermia in normal men. Combined administration of lower dosages of testosterone, similar to physiological replacement doses, plus a progestin or a GnRH analogue has demonstrated further suppression. Most of these male hormonal contraceptives have been associated with modest weight gain and suppression of serum high-density cholesterol levels.[3] The method has not been tested on adolescents.

OTHER CONTRACEPTIVE METHODS

Finally, intrauterine devices are not in common use during adolescence. Unless a pregnancy has proceeded, barrier methods such as caps and diaphragms are not in use during adolescence. Unfortunately, many adolescents have unprotected intercourse or use ineffective methods, such as periodic abstinence or coitus interruptus (withdrawal prior to ejaculation) (Table 8.1). The Pearl index of these methods may be as high as 16. This is why abortion remains so frequent during adolescence.

COMMENT

Psychological and social problems are common every time a young girl has an unwanted pregnancy. Informing young people about contraception is a responsibility of parents, teachers, physicians, reporters, etc. The theory that sex education and the promotion of contraception use encourages sexual activities is

Table 8.1 Contraceptive methods (%) used during adolescence in European countries, age 12–18 years[35]

Country	PA/CI	COCs	IUD	Barrier	Other/ no prophylaxis
Belgium	4.0	61.0	0	12.0	23.0
Denmark	NA	64.0	2.0	19.0	15.0
Finland	NA	32.0	0	50.0	18.0
France	NA	17.3	0.1	NA	NA
Germany	50.0	40.0	0	10.0	NA
Greece	30.5	40.5	3.8	20.7	4.5
Hungary	60.0	35.0	0	5.0	NA
Italy	39.2	7.9	0	31.2	NA
Netherlands	7.0	56.0	0	29.0	8.0
UK	3.0	43.0	1.0	5.0	48.0

PA/CI, periodic abstinence/coitus interruptus; COCs, combined oral contraceptives; IUD, intrauterine device; NA, information not available

incorrect. Teenagers have identified the main source of information concerning contraception as friends and the media. This is due to communication problems between parents and children. In Sweden, family and sex education are taught in schools and abortions are legal on demand, free contraceptive counselling is easily available at well-organised family planning units and youth health centres. Condoms and COCs are available at low cost and emergency contraception is sold over the counter. The above factors have resulted in a low teenage childbearing rate. In cases where the adolescent chooses to continue her pregnancy, the clinicians should remain available for further discussion during the pregnancy. If the adolescent chooses to present the child for adoption or to terminate her pregnancy, the gynaecologists should be available to provide for her subsequent health care and emotional support together with a psychologist. In either case, the clinicians should encourage the adolescent to continue her education and be available to help her identify appropriate community programmes. The organisation of family planning centres for adolescents is undoubtedly necessary and must become a governmental priority.

References

1. American Academy of Pediatrics Committee on Adolescence 1999 Adolescent pregnancy—current trends and issues 1998. Pediatrics 103(2):516–520
2. American Academy of Pediatrics Committee on Public Education 2001 Sexuality, contraception and the media. Pediatrics 107(1):191–194
3. Anawalt B D, Amory J K 2001 Advances in male hormonal contraception. Annals of Medicine 33(9):587–595
4. Brown J D, Greenberg B S, Buerkel-Rothfuss N L 1993 Mass media, sex, and sexuality. Adolescent Medicine 4:511–525
5. Creatsas G, Guerrero E, Guilbert E, Drouin J, Serfaty D, Lemieux L, Suissa S, Colin P 2001 A multinational evaluation of the efficacy, safety and acceptability of the Protectaid contraceptive sponge. European Journal of Contraception and Reproductive Health Care 6:172–182

6. Creatsas G, Kontopoulou-Griva I, Deligeoroglou E, Digenopoulou L, Tsangaris A, Kallipolitis G, Milingos S, Michalas S 1997 Effect of the monophasic and triphasic (gestodene-ethinylestradiol) oral contraceptives on natural inhibitor and other haemostatic variables. The European Journal of Contraception and Reproductive Health Care 2(1):31–38

7. Creatsas G, Vekemans M, Horejsi J et al 1995 Adolescent sexuality in Europe. Multicentric study, International Federation of Infantile and Juvenile Gynecology. Adolescent Pediatrics and Gynecology 8:59–63

8. Creatsas G 2004 Contraception for adolescents 2003. In: Sultan C (ed) Pediatric and adolescent gynecology: evidence-based clinical practice. Karger, Basel, pp 225–232

9. Creatsas G 1997 Improving adolescent sexual behavior a tool for better fertility outcome and safe motherhood. International Journal of Obstetrics and Gynecology 58:85–92

10. Croxatto H B 2002 Progestin implants for female contraception. Contraception 65:15–19

11. Deligeoroglou E, Michailidis E, Creatsas G 2003 Oral contraceptives and reproductive system cancer. Annals of the New York Academy of Sciences 997:199–208

12. Deligeoroglou E 1997 Dysfunctional uterine bleeding. Annals of the New York Academy of Sciences 816:158–164

13. Deligeoroglou E 2000 Dysmenorrhea. Annals of the New York Academy of Sciences 900:237–244

14. Edgardh K 2002 Adolescent sexual health in Sweden. Sexually Transmitted Infections 78(5):352–356

15. Ellertson C, Trussell J, Stewart F, Koenig J, Raymond E G, Shochet T 2001 Emergency contraception. Seminars in Reproductive Medicine 19(4):323–330

16. Goldman J A, Dicker D, Feldberg D, Samuel N, Resnik R 1985 Barrier contraception in the teenager a comparison of four methods in adolescent girls. Adolescent Pediatrics and Gynecology 3:59–76

17. Haffner D W (ed) 1995 Facing facts: sexual health for America's adolescents. The Report of the National Commission on Adolescent Sexual Health. Sexuality Information and Education Council of the United States, New York

18. Hatcher R A, Trussell J, Stewart F et al 1998 Contraceptive technology, 17th edn. Ardent Media, New York

19. Heard-Dimyan J 1999 Issue of emergency hormonal contraception through a casualty department in a community hospital. British Journal of Family Planning 25(3):105–109

20. Institute of Medicine, Committee on Prevention and Control of Sexually Transmitted Diseases 1997 In: Eng T R, Butler W T (eds) The hidden epidemic. National Academy Press, Washington, DC (Centers for Disease Control and Prevention [CDC], 2000)

21. Jordan T R, Price J H, Fitzgerald S 2000 Rural parents' communication with their teenagers about sexual issues. Journal of School Health. 70(8):338–344

22. Kuyoh M A, Toroitich-Ruto C, Grimes D A, Schulz K F, Gallo M G 2004 Sponge versus diaphragm for contraception (Cochrane Review). The Cochrane Library, Issue 1. Update Software, Oxford

23. Manning W D, Longmore M A, Giordano P C 2000 The relationship context of contraceptive use at first intercourse. Family Planning Perspectives 32(3): 104–110

24. Ott M A, Adler N E, Millstein S G, Tschann J M, Ellen J M 2002 The trade-off between hormonal contraceptives and condoms among adolescents. Perspectives on Sexual and Reproductive Health 34(1):6–14

25. Paukku M, Quan J, Darney P, Raine T 2003 Adolescents' contraceptive use and pregnancy history: is there a pattern? Obstetrics and Gynecology 101(3):534–538

26. Roberts D F, Foehr U G, Rideout V J, Brodie M 1999 Kids and media at the new millennium: a comprehensive national analysis of children's media use. Henry J. Kaiser Family Foundation, Menlo Park, CA

27. Roper Starch Worldwide Inc 1999 The America online/Roper Starch youth cyberstudy. http://corp.aol.com/press/study/youthstudy.pdf

28. Schuster M A, Bell R M, Berry S H, Kanouse D E 1998 Impact of a high school condom availability program on sexual attitudes and behaviors. Family Planning Perspectives 30:67–72, 88

29. Sonenstein F L, Ku L C, Lindberg L D, Turner C F, Pleck J H 1998 Changes in sexual behavior and condom use among teenage males: 1988 to 1995. American Journal of Public Health 88:956–959

30. Spruyt A, Steiner M J, Joanis C et al 1998 Identifying condom users at risk for breakage and slippage: findings from three

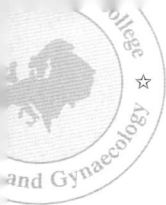

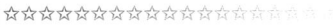

international sites. American Journal of Public Health 88:239–244

31. Stewart F H, Harper C C, Ellertson C E, Grimes D A, Sawaya G F, Trussell J 2001 Clinical breast and pelvic examination requirements for hormonal contraception: current practice vs. evidence. Journal of the American Medical Association 285(17):2232–2239

32. Strasburger V C 1993 Adolescents and the media: five crucial issues. Adolescent Medicine 4:479–493

33. Van Damme L 2000 Advances in topical microbicides. Paper presented at XIII International AIDS Conference, July 9–14, Durban, South Africa

34. Ventura S J, Mosher W D, Curtin S C, Abma J C, Henshaw S 2000 Trends in pregnancies and pregnancy rates by outcome: estimates for the United States, 1976–96. Vital Health Statistics 21 56:1–47

35. Wanner M S, Couchenour R L 2002 Hormonal emergency contraception. Pharmacotherapy 22(1):43–53

9

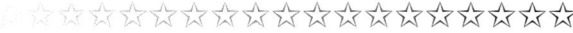
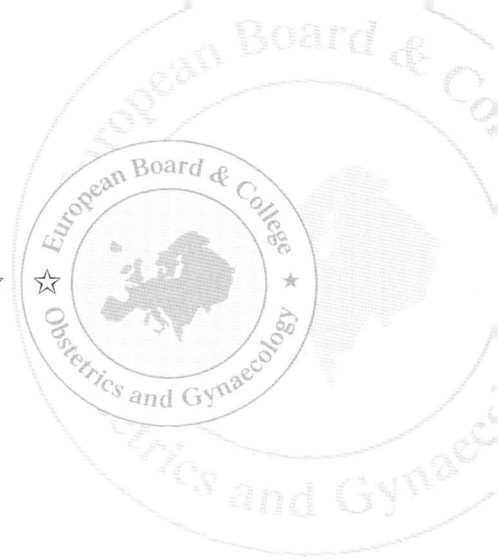

Contraception for the premenopausal woman

Vit Unzeitig

ABSTRACT

This chapter characterises the premenopausal period and reviews pregnancy implications and contraceptive options for women over 40 years of age. The information provided is based on an extensive literature review.

There are trends in the industrialised part of the world to postpone pregnancy to later in life. Premenopause (defined as the period over 40 years of age) is characterised by a progressive loss of ovarian function with/without dysfunctional uterine bleeding. However, premenopausal women are still potentially fertile and pregnancy in this phase of life is associated with an increased miscarriage rate, fetal anomalies and perinatal risks. Contraception at this age has special risks and benefits, both should be balanced to choose between available options. Each contraceptive method and its suitability in the premenopause are discussed, with an emphasis on modern combined oral contraception. Therefore, for women with certain risk factors, sterilisation, barrier methods, progestin-only methods and intrauterine devices could be better choices.

Conclusion:

- contraception in the premenopause improves quality of life and prevents certain serious diseases;
- the variety of contraceptive options demands individual counselling and compliance;
- the risk of cardiovascular disease of any description is low in COC users;
- women can minimise their arterial risks by not smoking and by having their blood pressure checked before using a COC;
- users may decrease their venous thromboembolic risk by their choice of COC preparation although the effects will be modest.

KEYWORDS

Contraception, reproduction, premenopause, intrauterine device, risks, benefits

143

INTRODUCTION

With the increase in the average age of menopause, the reproductive period during which a woman can become pregnant and during which there is the necessity to effectively prevent pregnancy has been prolonged. In Europe, menopause usually occurs between the age of 46 and 54 years, and the question is: at which age should we speak of contraception in the later reproductive period? From the perspective of hormonal contraception, the traditional boundary has been 35 years, after which hormonal contraception was previously not recommended at all. Although today this boundary remains for combined oral contraception (COC) in women smokers, from the biological and social perspective, the age of 40 years presents itself as a better boundary, when the biological changes characteristic of the premenopause may begin to occur. In eastern European countries, in recent years, we have observed the trend seen in advanced countries, which is the postponement of pregnancy to a later age. From this stems the fact that we can consider a woman's reproductive functions to be fulfilled after 40 years of age. Therefore, in the following text, we will consider women older than 40 years, and for this period we will use the term premenopause, although in many women of this age a fully functional ovarian cycle may be preserved.

CHARACTERISTICS OF PREMENOPAUSE

From the biological perspective, this period is characterised by the progressive loss of ovarian function. First, there is luteal insufficiency, which leads to a relative abundance of estrogens. During this time, a regular monophasic anovulatory cycle may be preserved, but there may also be the first occurrences of dysfunctional uterine bleeding. The greatest number of curettages and hysterectomies (and possibly endometrial ablations) performed for the indication of menometrorrhagia fall into the period of the premenopause. With the decrease in estrogen levels below that necessary for endometrial proliferation, menopause occurs (the period of the last menstrual cycle) and postmenopause begins. Postmenopause is characterised by a hypergonadotrophic state with the gradual development of the climacteric syndrome. With increased levels of gonadotropins during the decrease in estrogens before the menopause, we may observe the symptoms of the climacteric syndrome even in the premenopause. This fact will certainly influence our therapeutic approach in the choice of method of contraception.

From the perspective of reproduction, this period has distinct characteristics. In women over 40 years, most pregnancies are unplanned and a large percentage are terminated by spontaneous or therapeutic abortion (Table 9.1).

Besides the risks associated with abortion, there are also the possible risks of delivery. Above 40 years of age, maternal mortality is four-times greater than in the group under age 30, and perinatal mortality almost doubles with the doubling of maternal age.

Table 9.1 Abortions by category and age of the women per 100 births in the Czech Republic in 2003

Age	Spontaneous	Legally-induced	Ectopic pregnancies	Total abortions
30–34	12.29	28.56	1.76	42.66
35–39	22.46	72.21	2.91	97.70
40–44	54.62	186.24	4.52	245.68
45–49	164.29	495.24	9.52	669.05

Although the probability of conception gradually decreases after 35 years of age, with respect to the fluctuating hormone levels, the risk of pregnancy remains for up to one year after menopause. If menopause occurs before 45 years, we should consider the risk of pregnancy for up to two years. Pregnancy may even occur when symptoms of the climacteric syndrome are present. Overall, fertility in this period is characterised by extreme individual variability.

THE REQUIREMENTS FOR CONTRACEPTION IN PREMENOPAUSE

Besides the requirements for contraception during the entire female reproductive period, which on the most basic level can be characterised as safety and reliability, in the premenopause there are specific requirements and certain qualities of individual methods of contraception gain significance. Conversely, certain adverse effects of various methods of contraception have a substantially decreased significance in premenopause than in younger age groups—for example, the generally decreased incidence of STDs in this age category and thus also a decreased incidence of inflammatory complications of IUDs.

In the ideal case, contraception for women in the premenopause should:

- be sufficiently effective;
- improve the quality of sexual life, which refers to maintaining a regular menstrual cycle and the estrogenic effect on overall appearance, libido, and the vaginal mucosa;
- eliminate climacteric symptoms—vasomotor, psychological, and somatic;
- eliminate problems associated with the menstrual cycle—premenstrual syndrome, irregular or painful menses, menorrhagia;
- decrease the incidence or manifestation of gynaecological diseases—pelvic inflammatory diseases (PID), extrauterine pregnancy, myomas, dysfunctional uterine bleeding, endometriosis, ovarian cysts, and not least gynaecological malignancies—in decreasing the incidence of these diseases, we also decrease the subsequent risks of their therapy, including repeated dilation, curettage and hysterectomy;
- ensure the prevention of osteoporosis;
- not mask the beginning of postmenopause;
- be devoid of adverse systemic effects, especially the influence on serious cardiovascular diseases, and not increase the risk of their development.

With respect to the constantly more frequent postponement of pregnancy to higher age categories, even during this period we cannot forget to consider the reversibility of individual methods and their effect on later fertility.

METHODS OF CONTRACEPTION AND THEIR SUITABILITY FOR THE PREMENOPAUSE

NATURAL METHODS

These methods are based on the estimation of the date of ovulation and the limited time of the ability of human gametes to become fertilised. In view of the hormonal dysbalance and frequent irregularities of the menstrual cycle during premenopause, these methods are completely inappropriate.

BARRIER METHODS

Decreased fertility and the decreased frequency of intercourse (mostly in monogamous relationships) significantly aid the reliability of barrier methods in the period of premenopause. There are male contraceptive methods (the condom) and female methods (the diaphragm), best in combination with spermicides. Barrier contraception is devoid of adverse systemic effects and its only serious disadvantage besides possibly decreased sensitivity is the necessity of application just prior to intercourse. If the sexual partners have prior experience with this method of contraception, then we recommend its use even in premenopause. In new users, we expect less reliability due to possible user error and decreased comfort and satisfaction. At every age, the reliability and satisfaction of users is dependent on careful counselling from medical personnel.

SPERMICIDES

The most common spermicide, nonoxynol-9, is available either in the form of vaginal suppositories, foam or cream. Vaginal suppositories may be used alone, while cream is mostly intended for use in combination with a diaphragm. During the period of normal fertility, we do not recommend the use of spermicides alone for their decreased reliability (Pearl index 5–20), but in the premenopause we can consider their use. The combination of barrier methods and chemical contraception (for example a vaginal pessary impregnated with spermicide for single use) effectively reduces the risk of sexually transmitted diseases and, of course, the risk of the failure (Pearl index 4–7).

COMBINED ORAL CONTRACEPTIVES

For several years, estrogen-gestagen oral contraceptives (COCs) were considered taboo over 35 years of age. This was due to the increased risk of myocardial infarction and stroke, as well as thromboembolic disease in those using pills with an estrogen content several times greater than is common today. The results of epidemiological studies and views regarding this problem have gone through a certain development and we will return to them later.

Beneficial effects of estrogen-gestagen contraceptives

Let us first look at the beneficial effects of COCs in general and which of these effects are especially important in premenopause:

- high reliability, complete reversibility, and a protective influence on later fertility;
- protection against endometrial and ovarian carcinoma (this positive effect is probably the most important, and will be discussed in relation to hormonal contraception and malignancies);
- decreased incidence of benign tumours of the breast;
- decreased incidence of uterine myomas;
- regular menstrual cycle with decreased blood loss and decreased incidence of dysmenorrhoea;
- prevention of dysfunctional uterine bleeding;
- decreased incidence of ectopic pregnancy;
- decreased incidence of pelvic inflammatory disease;
- decreased incidence of ovarian cysts;
- prevention of increased bone resorption and thus prevention of osteoporosis;
- decreased incidence of endometriosis.

Some authors still state other suspected beneficial effects, but those listed above can be considered as seriously confirmed. Prevention of ovarian[3] and endometrial[8] carcinoma has an essential significance. The protective influence remains even after termination of contraceptive use. By decreasing the incidence of dysfunctional uterine bleeding and uterine myomas, we also decrease the subsequent risks of their therapy. In this we find a very significant potential of combined oral contraceptives, especially in the period of premenopause. Besides other beneficial effects, in this period, prevention of osteoporosis is also important.

Adverse effects of estrogen-gestagen contraceptives

In the selection of contraception in general, and especially in considering combined estrogen-gestagen contraceptives, besides the beneficial effects we are also mainly interested in adverse effects and contraindications. We can divide adverse effects into:

- cardiovascular disease—myocardial infarction, cerebral ischaemic attacks or cerebral haemorrhage, hypertension and thromboembolic disease;
- hepatic disease—hepatocellular adenoma and carcinoma, cholestatic jaundice, and gallstones;
- a possible influence on certain kinds of malignancies.

The first wide-ranging studies demonstrated an almost three- to five-fold increased risk of developing cardiovascular disease in users of estrogen-gestagen

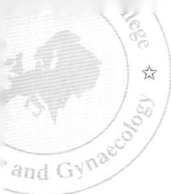

contraceptives. However, in these studies the women were primarily users of a pill with 50 or more micrograms of ethinylestradiol. Meta-analysis of studies from the 1980s, performed by Katerndahl et al,[6] demonstrated a significantly increased relative risk (RR) of thromboembolic disease (RR = 2.8), stroke (RR = 1.8), and myocardial infarction (RR = 1.6), while the overall mortality due to cardiovascular disease was not increased in contraceptive users (RR = 1.0).

We do not currently understand how COCs exert their cardiovascular effects. Modern COCs affect some aspects of haemostasis, lipoprotein, glucose and insulin metabolism and are also associated with small changes in blood pressure. Differences between preparations have been observed with respect to their effects on acquired resistance to activated protein C, with third generation COCs being more resistant than second generation ones.

The risk of cardiovascular disease is directly proportional to the dose of estrogens in the pill and significantly increases with smoking, especially above 15 cigarettes per day. In contrast, age alone in the absence of other risk factors practically does not increase this risk. At the beginning of the 1990s, it was generally accepted that for non-smokers there was no upper age limit in using combined hormonal contraceptives with ≤35 µg of ethinylestradiol, assuming that no other risk factors for cardiovascular disease were present. In his study[7] published in January 1996, Lewis states that the relative risk of myocardial infarction in users of contraceptives of the third generation is 1.1 with a confidence interval of 0.4–3.4. Statistically, this risk does not significantly differ from the risk in the control group of women without hormonal contraception. In the absence of a history of smoking and other conventional risk factors, current users of modern COCs probably do not have an increased risk of myocardial infarction.

Increased risk of ischaemic stroke (three- to four-fold greater than that among non-users) was found among all current users. This risk was not affected by duration of use. Higher relative risk in older users has been observed, perhaps because of changes in the prevalence of hypertension among older women. Greater relative risk has been observed among current users who smoke. Past use of COC has not been associated with a persisting elevated risk of ischaemic stroke—in some studies past users had a lower risk if compared with never users (any protective effect of COCs remains unclear).

Smoking and hypertension have often been found to be independent risk factors for haemorrhagic stroke. The risk of this event appeared to occur mostly in users aged 35 years or more. Relative risks of haemorrhagic stroke for all current COC users are 1.0–2.0, and have never been statistically significant. Also, there is no relationship with duration of use.

The wide-ranging epidemiological study,[10] focusing on the relationship between thromboembolic disease and combined contraceptives, aroused great interest in December 1995. This study of the World Health Organization consisted of 1143 users of contraceptives aged 20–44 years and 2998 controls from 21 centres in Africa, Asia, Europe, and Latin America. According to the WHO results, the use of contraceptives is associated with an increased risk of thromboembolic disease both in Europe (odds ratio 4.15) and developing countries (odds ratio 3.25). This risk is expressed within the first four months of use, and is not definitely influenced by age or by smoking. In contrast, a higher body mass index (above 25) is an independent risk factor of thromboembolic disease. Users of contraceptives with desogestrel or gestodene have a higher risk of thrombo-embolic disease than users of contraceptives containing levonorgestrel (odds ratio 2.6). The conclusions of these studies were analysed and confirmed in 2000.[5] Later, an increased risk of thromboembolic disease in users of contraceptives with cyproteron acetate has been discussed.[9] This risk probably exists.

In most contraceptive users, the estrogen component of the pill significantly increases the systolic and diastolic blood pressure. However, this increase is within the range of normal values and the mechanism is most likely the increased production of angiotensin and slight sodium retention. Still, regular blood pressure checks are the best screening methods for cardiovascular diseases even in normotensive users of oral contraceptives.

According to some studies the incidence of hepatic disease is higher in contraceptive users, but it remains at an extremely low level, and this risk is considerably counterbalanced by the beneficial effects of the contraceptives.[4] Furthermore, in these studies the women were mostly users of pills containing mestranol. The incidence of hepatocellular adenoma is approximately 1 case per 100 000 users in one year, and for hepatocellular carcinoma 3–4 cases per 1 000 000 users in one year. There is only a significantly increased incidence of cholecystolithiasis during the first few years of use, which provides evidence for the influence of pre-existing changes and thus is only an acceleration of their manifestation.

The following are the possible influences of estrogen-gestagen contraceptives on certain types of malignancies:

1. Breast cancer. Analysis of the results of many studies indicates a slightly increased relative risk (RR 1.5–2), but only for women who started using contraceptives at an early age, specifically before their first pregnancy, and who used contraceptives for a long period (8–12 years).

2. Endometrial carcinoma. There is a demonstrated decreased risk with contraceptive use >2 years (RR = 0.6) and >4 years (RR = 0.4).

3. Ovarian carcinoma. Decreased risk has also been demonstrated with use >4 years (RR = 0.5), and >7 years (RR = 0.2–0.3). In addition, the decreased risk remains even after termination of contraceptive use. With regard to the generally known difficulty in diagnosing ovarian carcinoma and the high mortality from the disease, this is evidently the most important beneficial effect of hormonal contraceptives.

4. Carcinoma of the cervix. Study results have been inconsistent, and methodological processing of data with regard to the proven association of the incidence of this disease with sexual behaviour has been difficult. There are studies that demonstrate a slightly increased risk, while many others have not confirmed this.[1] There are also doubts about the hormonal dependence of cervical cancer.

5. Malignant melanoma. It is impossible to infer definite conclusions because of the methodological difficulty in distinguishing contraceptive effects from the most significant risk factor, which is UV radiation. Nevertheless, there are studies demonstrating an increased risk of the disease after long-term use of the estrogen-progestin combination.[2]

Conditions for the prescription of estrogen-gestagen contraceptives

In conclusion, we can state that we prescribe combined oral contraceptives to women older than 35 years, under the following conditions:

- fundamentally a pill with ≤35 µg of ethinylestradiol;
- if possible a pill with gestagen with a very low androgenic activity (because of its influence on the lipids spectrum);
- strict regard for contraindications (even relative contraindications);
- normal liver enzymes, lipids, glycaemia, and mammography before prescription, and repeatedly negative results during regular examination every 12 months;
- prescription only to non-smokers and with the absence of other risk factors for cardiovascular disease;
- in the presence of climacteric problems and the need for contraception, rather select contraceptives than hormone replacement therapy, which does not have a sufficient contraceptive effect.

In keeping with these conditions the definition of the WHO is valid even for women older than 40 years: 'The use of combined oral contraceptives is generally safe and associated more with beneficial than adverse effects'.

PROGESTIN-ONLY CONTRACEPTIVES

This type of contraception is becoming more and more popular. We have the oral contraceptive form (desogestrel and lynestrenol), medroxyprogesterone acetate in the injectable form, and 3-ketodesogestrel (3-KDSG) or levonorgestrel in the form of subcutaneous implants. This type of contraception has certain advantages, which especially come to the forefront in the period of premenopause.

The advantages are:

- contraception with a high reliability;
- as yet non-existent epidemiological associations between gestagen-only contraceptives and an increased incidence of cardiovascular diseases or malignancies;
- protection against endometrial carcinoma;
- absence of adverse effects caused by estrogens;
- minimal influence on metabolic reactions;
- well tolerated even in women who did not tolerate combined estrogen-gestagen contraceptives.

In the period of the premenopause there is the added gestagenic protection of the hyperplastic endometrium during anovulatory cycles, which is reflected in the previously mentioned protection against endometrial carcinoma. The limiting factor of using this contraceptive during the pre- and perimenopause is the alteration in the menstrual cycle. During this period, metrorrhagia caused by gestagen-only contraceptives is indistinguishable from organic disease of the endometrium, and repeated curettage is not acceptable in this situation.

On the contrary, we can consider gestagen-only contraceptives with advantage when there are limits to the use of estrogens, for example in smokers over 35 years, in other contraindications of estrogens, in women with a predisposition to thromboembolic disease, diabetes mellitus, hypertension, migraine headaches, and they are very advantageous for overcoming the period of immobilisation after surgical procedures. From this point of view, contraceptive forms containing desogestrel (oral) or its metabolite 3-ketodesogestrel (implant) are very effective.

INTRAUTERINE CONTRACEPTION

The intrauterine device (IUD) is probably the most common type of contraception in women over 40 years in some European countries. It is among those methods with a high reliability and complete reversibility and, furthermore, it is not dependent on daily use or application just prior to intercourse. It has no serious systemic effects and, in this age group, the percentage of spontaneous expulsions or perforations is significantly decreased. In addition, due to the generally lower incidence of pelvic inflammatory disease in premenopause, the main adverse effect and contraindication of IUD is lessened. However, there may be serious adverse effects such as menorrhagia and irregular bleeding leading to curettage and extraction of the IUD. We certainly cannot expect control of the beginning of climacteric problems from the IUD, nor the beneficial influence on the incidence of dysfunctional uterine bleeding or malignancies. An IUD inserted after 40 years of age may be extracted up to one year after menopause, but sooner when uterine atrophy occurs.

The intrauterine system (IUS) with levonorgestrel is very effective. Levonorgestrel is released in a dose of 20 µg daily for a period of five years and has practically only a local effect on the endometrium and cervical mucus. The Pearl index ranges between 0 and 0.2, and the cumulative number of pregnancies for the entire five years is approximately 0.5–1.1% of users. Among the main advantages, besides high reliability, was a significant decrease in menstrual blood loss and also, in the period of premenopause, the very important prevention of endometrial hyperplasia during anovulatory cycles. With the physical changes of the cervical mucus, we can expect a decreased incidence of PID, not only in comparison with users of regular IUDs but also in comparison with the general population. There have also been reports of using the levonorgestrel IUS as a gestagen carrier in hormone substitution therapy in combination with any form of estradiol application.

POSTCOITAL CONTRACEPTION

Postcoital contraception does not have any specific characteristics in this age group and follows the same indications and contraindications as in the general population.

STERILISATION

In this age category, when irreversible contraception is desired, sterilisation is an appropriate method most probably without adverse effects and with a high reliability. The previously assumed acceleration of the occurrence of menopause has not been definitely proven. We cannot expect a beneficial influence on the menstrual cycle or on the climacteric syndrome. Even in this age group, there should be emphasis on careful counselling prior to the procedure to make it plain that the procedure is irreversible from the female perspective. In Europe, male sterilisation (vasectomy) is performed only sporadically.

CONLUSIONS

1. In the premenopause, the possibilities of modern contraception present not only an effective form of preventing pregnancy but also a means of preventing certain serious diseases.
2. With appropriate selection and use, contraceptives may significantly improve the woman's quality of life. In contrast, not respecting the limitations and contraindications of the individual methods can lead to the dissatisfaction of the user in the best case and damage to her health in the worst case.
3. The selection of contraception for this period requires a highly individualised approach to each woman, with a sound knowledge of the problems.
4. The arterial risks of COC can be minimised (and possibly removed entirely) by taking a careful personal and family history, and by checking the user's blood pressure. At all ages the effect of smoking on cardiovascular risk is greater than the effect of COC use.
5. The level of follicle stimulating hormone (FSH) higher than $40\,Uml^{-1}$ seems to be a marker for the stopping of a hormonal-contraceptive prescription.

References

1. Delgado-Rodriguez M, Sillero-Arenas M, Moreno-Martin J M et al 1992 Oral contraceptives and cancer of the cervix. A meta-analysis. Acta Obstetricia et Gynecologica Scandinavica 71:368–376
2. Feskanich D, Hunter D 1999 Oral contraceptive use and risk of melanoma in premenopausal women. British Journal of Cancer 81:918
3. Gross T P, Schlesselman J J 1994 The estimated effect of oral contraceptive use on the cumulative risk of epithelial ovarian cancer. Obstetrics and Gynecology 83:419–424
4. Hannaford P C, Kay C R, Vessey M P et al 1997 Combined oral contraceptives and liver disease. Contraception 55:145–151

5. Jick H, Kaye J A, Vasilakis-Scaramozza C, Jick S S 2000 Risk of venous thromboembolism among users of third generation oral contraceptives compared with users of oral contraceptives with levonorgestrel before and after 1995: cohort and case-control analysis. British Medical Journal 321:1190–1195

6. Katerndahl D A et al 1992 Cardiovascular diseases in users of estrogen-gestagen contraceptives. Journal of Family Practice 35:147–157

7. Lewis M A, Heinemann L A J, MacRae K D, Bruppacher R, Spitzer W O 1996 Transnational Research Group on Oral Contraceptives and the Health of Young Women: The increased risk of venous thromboembolism and the use of third generation progestagens: role of bias in observational research. Contraception 54:5–13

8. Schlesselman J J 1991 Oral contraceptives and neoplasia of the uterine corpus. Contraception 43:557–579

9. Vasilakis-Scaramozza C, Jick H 2001 Risk of venous thromboembolism with cyproterone or levonorgestrel contraceptives. Lancet 358:1427–1429

10. WHO Collaborative Study of Cardiovascular Disease and Steroid Hormone Contraception 1995 Venous thromboembolic disease and combined oral contraceptives: results of international multicentre case-control study. Lancet 346:1575–1582

10

☆☆☆☆☆☆☆☆☆☆☆☆☆☆☆☆☆ ☆

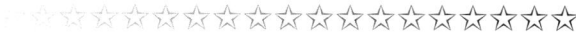

Sterilisation

László Kovács

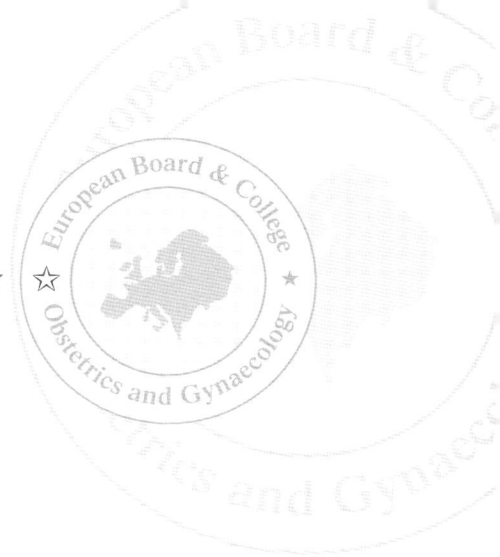

ABSTRACT

Voluntary sterilisation or voluntary surgical contraception has become an extremely popular and well-established contraceptive procedure, providing the most effective protection against pregnancy for couples who desire no more children. Compared with other methods of contraception, the advantages, which are equally applicable to tubal ligation and vasectomy, include the permanent nature of the procedure, the patient is not required to remember anything or interrupt sexual intercourse, and the procedure is cost-effective when the cost is spread out over time and it is highly effective in preventing pregnancy. The disadvantages include the permanent nature of the procedure (reversal is difficult and expensive), and the fact that no protection against sexually transmitted diseases is provided.

The technique of sterilisation mainly involves surgery: blocking of the Fallopian tubes in the female through laparoscopy, using electrocoagulation or mechanical devices (rings or clips), or through laparotomy by ligation and partial resection of the tubes, or vasectomy in the male through a small incision in the scrotum.

The failure rate over a ten-year follow-up is about 1%. Complications are rare. The mortality risk for the female is about 4 per 100 000 operations, half being due to complications from the general anaesthesia. Vasectomy is essentially not associated with mortality. The very few exceptions due to infections, most likely involve tetanus.

A small proportion of sterilised persons regret their infertility and request reversal. The success rate is higher in the male. In the female, it depends on the sterilisation technique—the less damaged the tubes, the better the chances. For the time being, in vitro fertilisation and embryo transfer promise the best results.

KEYWORDS

Voluntary surgical contraception, female, male, laparoscopic sterilisation, electrocoagulation, Falope ring, tubal clips, vasectomy, no-scalpel vasectomy, regret, reversal

INTRODUCTION

Currently, more than half (57%) of all couples in the world are protected from pregnancy by the use of contraceptives: 53% in the less developed and 72% in the more developed regions, a quarter of them having undergone sterilisation.[5] In a global context, sterilisation occupies first place among contraceptive methods.

Voluntary sterilisation or voluntary surgical contraception has become an extremely popular and well-established contraceptive procedure, providing the most effective protection against pregnancy for couples who desire no more children. It offers many advantages over other contraceptive methods because it is a once-only procedure that almost completely eliminates the risk of unwanted pregnancy and the sequelae of induced abortion. It does not entail regular check-ups and it eliminates the need for, or expense of, continued contraceptive supplies, making it very cost-effective. If the procedure is performed according to accepted medical standards, the risk of complications is small. The disadvantages of the two forms of sterilisation are: the permanent nature of the procedures (they are difficult and expensive to reverse), and the fact that they do not provide protection against sexually transmitted diseases.

A marked increase in contraceptive sterilisation began shortly after the introduction and rapid spreading of the use of oral contraceptives. It seems likely that experience with the pill was an important catalyst for the mass acceptance of sterilisation. Oral contraceptives introduced a dramatic change from the prior contraceptive regimen, because they were much more effective and because they separated contraception from sexual intercourse. However, as concerns about the long-term safety of oral contraceptives grew, tubal sterilisation and vasectomy became increasingly attractive as alternatives that shared the characteristics of being highly effective and safe.

Voluntary surgical contraception, however, presents certain problems that are not shared by other contraceptive methods. As it is a surgical procedure, it requires professional personnel, equipment and back-up facilities. Also, because surgical contraception results in permanent sterility, in certain countries it is still an object of fear, controversy and prejudice, and evokes political, cultural and religious objections. Although ongoing research may lead to the development of non-surgical methods, and while the reversibility of the procedures has been improved in recent years, at present the procedure should be considered to be both surgical and permanent.

Tubal sterilisation has become much more common than vasectomy: the global prevalence of female sterilisation is 17%, and that of male sterilisation 5%. In the developing countries the levels are 20% and 5%, while in the developed countries they are 8% and 4%, respectively. However, vasectomy is safer, less expensive, and equally effective in preventing pregnancies than other methods. This apparent paradox may have several explanations. One of them is the definitely higher motivation of women in fertility control; consequently, they find it easier to decide and to accept being sterilised. Furthermore, the proportion of unmarried women is increasing and they are increasingly choosing sterilisation.

The delusion that vasectomy will impair a man's sexual ability prevents many male partners from easily accepting sterilisation.

The performance of sterilisation naturally depends on the availability of services. Female surgical contraception requires an appropriate medical facility, because it is an abdominal operation. Section of the vas in the male depends on an aseptic minor surgical technique. The risks of complications and mortality are greater for women, and more equipment and emergency services are needed. Male surgical contraception is a minor procedure and complications are generally related to infection or bleeding beneath the skin.

LEGAL REGULATIONS

The laws governing surgical contraception vary widely from country to country. Three decades ago (but in some places even today), the legislation governing surgical contraception was highly restrictive and almost always related to pregnancy-related contraindications of a medical, obstetrical or genetic nature.

Today, this trend has changed. In most countries, surgical contraception is frequently performed at the request of the individual as a form of permanent contraception. In these countries, the legislation explicitly declares that voluntary surgical contraception is legal, or it is implicitly legal because no law prohibits it. In some countries, statutes or government decrees make voluntary surgical contraception a criminal offence. In some places, the legal status of voluntary surgical contraception is unclear.

Most legislations require an adequate time interval (30–90 days) between the counselling and the procedure itself, in order to permit a well-considered decision.

COUNSELLING

When the family size is considered to be complete or there is a specific medical contraindication to continuing fertility, then sterilisation becomes the contraceptive method of choice. It is essential to counsel both partners about the nature of the procedures and their implications and to discuss whether it is better for the male or female partner to be sterilised.

The answer usually depends on whichever partner is the more sure that no other pregnancies are desired. It must be kept in mind, however, that with present techniques female surgical contraception is more costly and more time-consuming and carries a slightly greater surgical risk than the male procedure of vasectomy.

Counselling should include a discussion of all contraceptive methods available, including their risks and benefits, with emphasis on the expected permanent nature of the procedure and a discussion of the surgical nature of the procedure and the types of anaesthesia available. Counselling should include reference to the failure rates and to the question of reversibility. A discussion of non-medical issues, such as lifestyle and future possibilities (e.g. the death of a living child, the possibilities of divorce and a new marriage, etc.), is also necessary.

FEMALE STERILISATION

INDICATIONS

Both contraceptive and medical reasons may serve as indications.

Contraceptive indications

Surgical contraception has become a widely accepted procedure for permanent contraception for couples who want no more children and have no other specific indication.

Medical indications

Medical indications for surgical contraception are defined as conditions that would make pregnancy hazardous. The indications are generally related only to surgical contraception of the woman, although a considerate man may choose to undergo surgical contraception in order to protect the woman.

Chronic systemic diseases are the most widely accepted medical indications for surgical contraception. These include chronic cardiac, pulmonary, renal, endocrine and other diseases.

Obstetrical indications may vary, from a definite history of obstetrical complications to high parity. For example, sterilisation is commonly used after multiple caesarean sections.

Surgical contraception may be required by individuals with a family history of heritable diseases, which are usually inherited as a recessive, but sometimes as a dominant strain.

Surgical contraception for the mentally handicapped has been a topic involving a great deal of controversy. The indications are too uncertain and the possibilities of abuse obvious. A mentally handicapped person unable to take care of herself is certainly unable to take care of any offspring. In addition, the use of temporary methods of contraception by mentally handicapped patients is difficult to ensure, and enforcement of abstinence is unlikely. The problem with surgically sterilising these patients is that the woman cannot give informed consent and the decision has to be delegated to the institution involved, to guardians, to parents or to a court. The lack of clear laws on this subject in many countries presents both the physician and the family with a difficult situation. The basic right of the individual must always be borne in mind.

TIMING OF THE OPERATION

Female surgical contraception may be carried out as an interval procedure, postpartum, at the time of an abortion or at the time of other pelvic surgery.

Interval surgical contraception

Interval surgical contraception may be performed at the convenience of the patient and the physician. The timing of the operation is best in the first half of the menstrual cycle. If this is not possible, then it is important to ascertain that the woman is not pregnant.

In one study, the women underwent a pre-operative pregnancy assessment test on a fasting morning urine sample on the day of planned surgery. Of the 802 women admitted, 21 (2.6%) were found to be pregnant.[9]

Laparoscopic sterilisation is a high-risk area for potential litigation in gynaecological practice. It is recommended that a pregnancy test be performed on each case of laparoscopic sterilisation as a routine procedure during the immediate pre-operative assessment.

Postpartum sterilisation

Whenever possible, a woman's decision should be made a reasonable amount of time before delivery and not during the emotional stress of labour. Postpartum surgical contraception is performed immediately, or at most a few days after delivery. At the thinned abdominal wall, the separation of the rectus muscles and the enlarged uterus permit access to the Fallopian tubes through a very small incision made at the level of the tubes, high in the abdomen. When carried out at this time, the procedure scarcely increases the length of the hospital stay after delivery. Postpartum surgical contraception has no effect on either the quantity or the composition of the breast milk.

Sterilisation at the time of an abortion

Surgical contraception can be performed at the time of an abortion. However, it is important to ensure that the decision is not made under the emotional stress of the abortion.

Sterilisation at the time of other pelvic surgery

When a caesarean section is to be performed, the surgeon should have formal permission in advance to perform tubal occlusion if this appears indicated. Some gynaecological operations, such as the removal of an ovarian cyst or plastic vaginal repair, may also be accompanied by a surgical contraception if indications exist.

SURGICAL APPROACHES

As for most surgery involving the internal reproductive organs, the route to the surgical area may be through either the abdomen or the vagina.

The abdominal route

Minilaparotomy

For the generally trained gynaecologist, the abdominal incision is simplest and furnishes the most unobstructed exposure of the tubes.

Postpartum ligation and section of the tubes has been practised through a very small lower midline incision.

In the non-puerperal woman, a similarly short incision (less than 5 cm) can be used. This procedure, which employs a suprapubic incision, is called a mini-laparotomy. With such an incision in the not recently pregnant woman, the tubes must be brought to an anterior position, by using a uterine elevator inserted vaginally into the uterine cavity.

Operative techniques

The Madlener technique. In the Madlener technique, the simplest of all methods, a loop of tube is picked up with forceps and a crushing clamp is placed across both limbs of the loop. A non-absorbable suture is then tied over the crushed area. In a modification of this technique, the intervening segment may be resected (Figs 10.1A, B).

The Pomeroy technique. The Pomeroy technique differs from the modified Madlener technique only in that a plain catgut ligature is tied about the two limbs of the loop without prior crushing. The intervening segment is then resected (Figs 10. 2A–D).

The Irving technique. The Irving technique was devised to provide further protection against reopening of the proximal segment. In this method, the proximal and distal segments of the transected tube are separated by drawing the end of the proximal part through a surgically created myometrial tunnel in the anterior or posterior wall of the uterus and anchoring it there.

The vaginal approach

Vaginal approaches, such as colpotomy or culdoscopy, may be associated with a higher incidence of major complications than the abdominal route, including post-operative pelvic infection, and are much less frequently used.

Laparoscopy

If the sterilisation is performed as an interval procedure, laparoscopy is generally used. The laparoscope is inserted through a subumbilical incision. In modern laparoscopes, optical and surgical elements have been combined in a single instrument

A   B

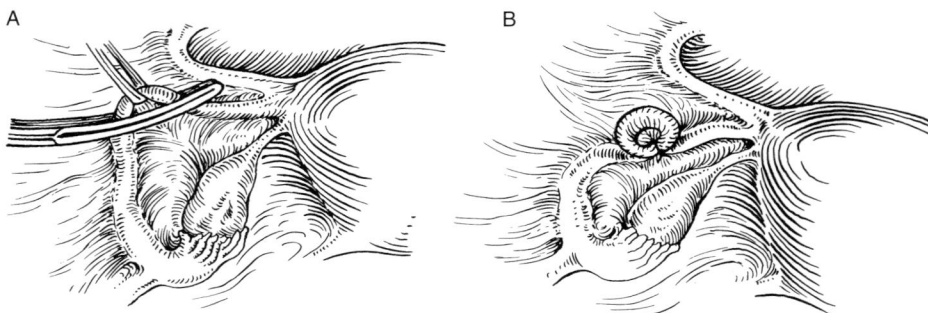

Fig 10.1 Madlener technique of tubal occlusion.
A, crushing of the tube; **B**, ligature of the tube. (With permission from the author[10])

Contraception and family planning

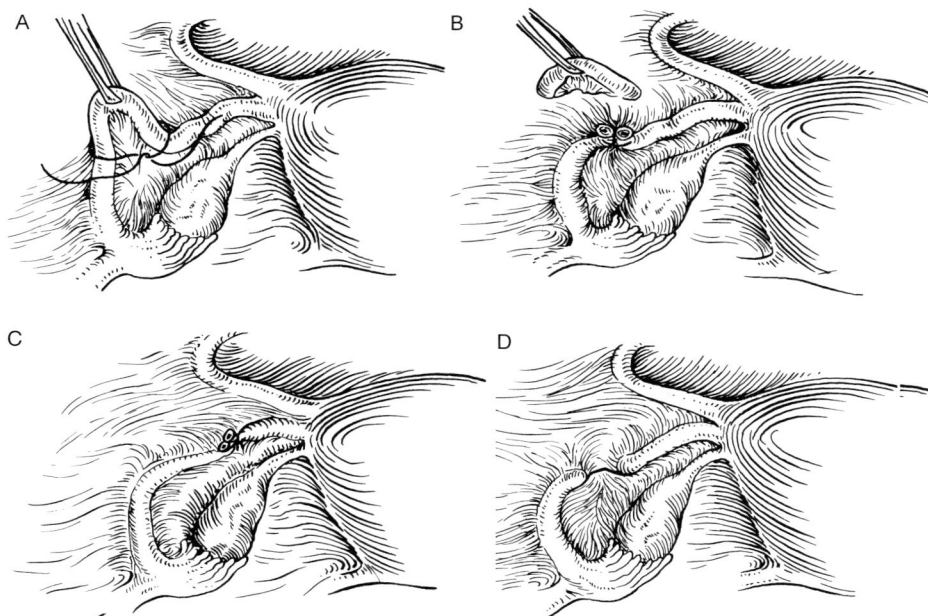

Fig 10.2 Pomeroy technique of tubal occlusion.
A, ligature; **B**, resection of the loop; **C**, completed surgery; **D**, situation after healing. (With permission from the author[10])

that needs only one abdominal puncture (Fig 10.3). After identification of the tubes, either they are grasped and electrocoagulated, or bands or clips are applied.

Electrocoagulation

Electrocoagulation is a method that has been developed to interrupt the Fallopian tube in the laparoscopic approach. The isthmus of the tube is grasped by special electrocoagulation forceps and an electric current is applied to the tube to coagulate a segment about 3–4 cm in length (Fig 10.4). The electric current may be unipolar or bipolar. Unipolar current enters through the forceps and leaves through a moistened lead electrode plate placed on the patient's thigh. Bipolar electric current enters and leaves through the two ends of the forceps, and is therefore much safer. Accidental burning of the bowel or other adjacent structures is a real risk with any of the electrical methods.

Mechanical devices

Rings and clips are commonly used in the laparoscopic approach, but can also be applied in minilaparotomy, colpotomy and culdoscopy. They are popular because of the avoidance of accidental electrical burns, the diminished likelihood of subsequent ectopic pregnancy and, in the case of the clips, the minimal degree of tubal destruction, which allows maximum reversibility.

Rings. The Falope ring, a silicone rubber band, has recently been extensively used.[24] A special applicator is used to grasp a loop of the isthmic portion of the

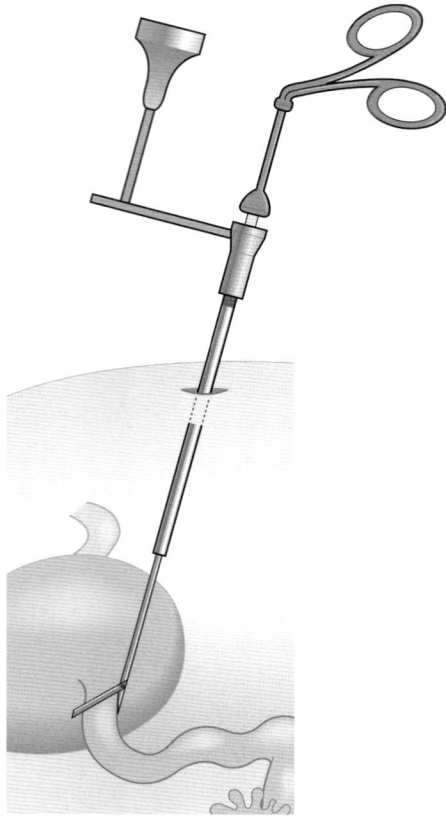

Fig 10.3 Laparoscopic sterilisation using the operating laparoscope. (With permission from the authors[6])

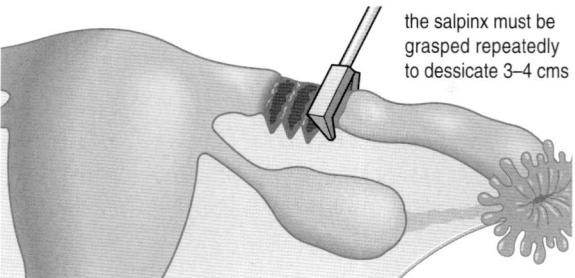

the salpinx must be grasped repeatedly to dessicate 3–4 cms

Fig 10.4 Bipolar electrocoagulation.
The salpinx must be grasped repeatedly to desiccate 3–4 cm. (With permission from the authors[6])

tube and to slip the ring on to its base (Figs 10.5A–E), where it tightly constricts, cutting off the circulation to the loop of the Fallopian tube. This causes tissue necrosis, followed by healing and fibrosis, leading to permanent tubal occlusion.

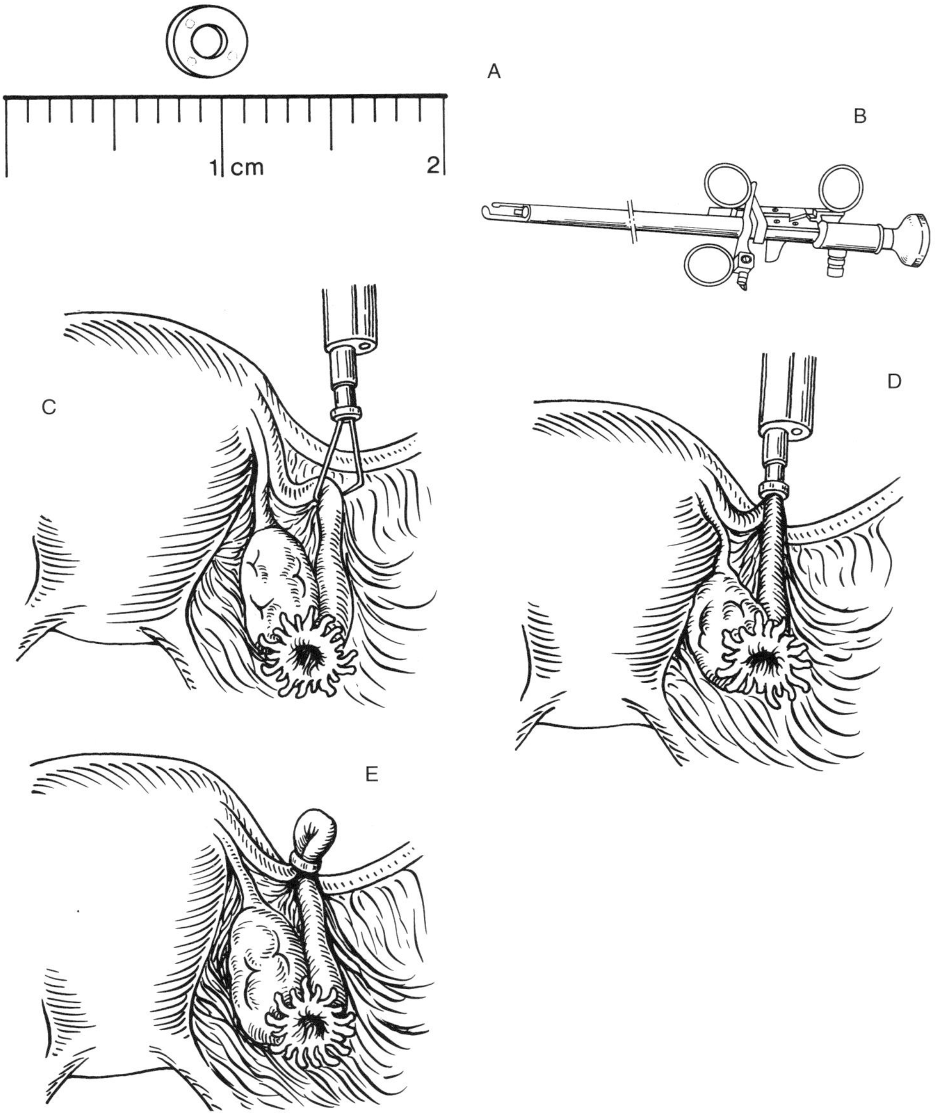

Fig 10.5 **A**, Yoon ring; **B**, applicator; **C**, lifting the tube; **D**, application of the ring; **E**, completed occlusion. (With permission from the author[10])

Clips. A number of occlusive clips have been developed to provide a method for inflicting minimal damage to the tube, so as to enhance the potential for reversibility. The Filshie clip has an outer surface of titanium and a soft-ridged inner core of Silastic®. The Filshie clip is believed to have an advantage in that it is able to accommodate oedematous tubes often found in postpartum cases. With the use of a Filshie clip, only the part of the tube that is compressed between the jaws of the clip (about 4 mm) is damaged.

The Hulka-Clemens spring-loaded clip has two plastic-toothed jaws hinged by a metal pin and locked around the tubes by a stainless steel spring (Figs 10.6A, B).

Bands and clips obviate the use of electrocoagulation in the laparoscopic approach and inflict less damage on the Fallopian tube, while achieving the same effectiveness. They preserve more tubal length, so reversal is more possible.

Following laparoscopy, patients usually need only a short stay in the hospital. They will have approximately one hour to recover from the general anaesthesia and will then be sent home. A patient will usually be given 24 hours to recover post-operatively before returning to work.

Post-operative instructions for tubal ligations include resting for 24 hours after surgery, the taking of analgesics as needed for pain relief, no bathing for 48 hours post-operatively, and the avoidance of sexual intercourse and strenuous lifting for one week in order to allow the incision to heal.

BLIND DELIVERY SYSTEMS

Non-surgical sterilisation has the potential of being a simple, inexpensive and well-accepted procedure. One non-surgical approach involves the use of

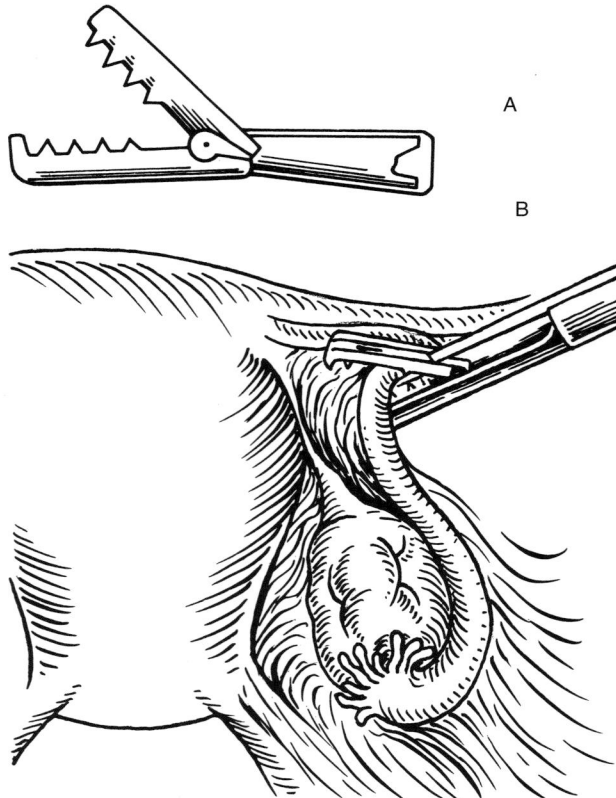

A

B

Fig 10.6 A, Hulka clip; **B**, clip application. (With permission from the author[10])

quinacrine pellets to produce occlusion of the Fallopian tubes. The most commonly used regimen, first described by Zipper et al,[25] involves the introduction of seven 36 mg pellets of quinacrine hydrochloride into the uterus by a modified IUD inserter during two separate insertions one month apart. Although quinacrine has not been approved for clinical use as a method of sterilisation by any drug regulatory agency in the developed world it has been used in numerous countries, most probably in several hundreds of thousands of women. Efficacy and safety analyses have been reported from Vietnam[20,21] and Chile.[7] The cumulative pregnancy probabilities were about 5–6 per 100 women five years after the treatment and about 10 per 100 women after ten years. A marked difference was demonstrable, depending on age: those aged below 35 years at the sterilisation treatment had about 11 pregnancies per 100 women, while those aged above 35 had only three.

The contraceptive effectiveness of quinacrine pellets is lower than that of surgical sterilisation or the modern IUDs. Nonetheless, it is a reasonably effective alternative among older recipients and it avoids the risk of surgery and the side effects of IUDs.

In recent years, several groups of experts have discussed the safety and efficacy of quinacrine sterilisation. Numerous concerns have been expressed: the effectiveness was questionable because of the widely varying pregnancy rates; on the basis of the published data, the long-term safety, side effects and complications could not be adequately assessed; and because of the suspected mutagenic effects of the drug, studies were needed to examine whether quinacrine could cause cancer or malformations in the fetus in cases of contraceptive failures. For the time being it is recommended that, until the above concerns have been properly investigated, quinacrine should not be offered to women as a method of sterilisation.[8]

Another approach of non-surgical tubal occlusion involves placing plugs into the Fallopian tubes. Silicone instillation during hysteroscopy (Ovabloc®) is possible in about 90% of the candidates. The position of the plugs needs to be checked later by means of ultrasonography because expulsion either to the abdomen or to the uterine cavity may occur in about 6% of cases. In a study with observation for 18 393 months of exposure, the cumulative pregnancy rate was 0.99. The uses of Ovabloc® should be limited to women who will benefit from a less invasive sterilisation method, although it should be remembered that there is a risk of primary failure and the expulsion of successfully instilled silicones.[12]

EFFECTIVENESS

The effectiveness of surgical sterilisation is measured by pregnancy rates. Luteal-phase pregnancy is defined as conception occurring immediately before surgery, and method failures are defined as conceptions subsequent to sterilisation. Failure rates vary with the method, the timing of surgery and the age of the woman. Pregnancies after sterilisation are more often ectopic, and ectopic rates also vary with the sterilisation method.

Contraception and family planning

Many early studies reported failure rates of <1%. Because of the brief or incomplete follow-up, such low failure rates are now recognised to be underestimates. The Collaborative Review of Sterilisation (CREST)[15] study identified a ten-year cumulative failure rate of 18.5 per 1000 for all methods combined.

Pregnancies occurring after sterilisation are more likely to be ectopic than are pregnancies occurring in an unsterilised population. The CREST study demonstrated a ten-year cumulative probability of ectopic pregnancy of 7.3 per 1000 women for all methods combined.

The effectiveness of bipolar electrocoagulation through laparoscopy is highly dependent on the surgical technique. In one survey, women who had fewer than three sites of coagulation had a failure probability of 12.9 per 1000 procedures. By contrast, women who had three or more sites coagulated had a probability of failure of 3.2 per 1000 procedures.

It can be concluded that the long-term probability of pregnancy after tubal sterilisation with bipolar coagulation was very low when three or more sites of the Fallopian tube were coagulated. Bipolar coagulating systems can be highly effective for sterilisation when the Fallopian tubes are adequately coagulated.[16]

COMPLICATIONS OF FEMALE STERILISATION

Early complications

Female surgical contraception may be associated with complications similar to those of any gynaecological procedure involving minimal manipulation but requiring opening of the peritoneum. The majority of these complications are of a minor nature.

The lowest rate is observed with laparoscopy (0.9–1.7%), laparotomy has approximately twice the risk of complications. The most common complication arises when there is a need to convert a laparoscopic procedure to a laparotomy because of the inability to complete the sterilisation laparoscopically, with most studies demonstrating a 1% incidence. This complication is caused by adhesions from previous surgery in over two-thirds of the cases. Other laparoscopic surgical complications include mesosalpingeal tears and transection of the tube, which may require laparotomy to control bleeding (up to 0.6%).

Bowel burns can occur from accidental electrocoagulation, resulting in late perforation and peritonitis (up to 0.6%). Both with laparoscopy and with laparotomy, there is always a chance of wound infection and/or breakdown (1%).

The mortality risk is 3.6 to 4.0 per 100 000 tubal ligation procedures, with one half being due to complications from the general anaesthesia, and the other half due to the operative procedure.

Late sequelae

The psychological effects of the operation have received considerable study. The great majority of women continue to be satisfied with the operation, but a minority experience feelings of regret or may 'feel different' in a psychological way after their operation.

Psychosocial issues regarding sterilisation can be divided into three major areas: issues of regret, psychological or psychiatric problems, and sexual satisfaction.

A number or studies have looked at possible factors that would predict those at risk of regret. Unfortunately, these studies have all differed in their definition of regret, which was taken to mean anything ranging from other than being completely satisfied to seeking reversal of the procedure. In the studies by Abraham et al[1] and Taylor et al,[22] the definition of regret included only those women who sought reversal. The individuals seeking reversal were younger at the time of operation, were more likely to be sterilised at their partner's request, and were more likely to have entered a new marriage.

In the collaborative review of sterilisation (CREST study[23]), which consisted of a multicentre, prospective observational study, 2 and 2.7% of the more than 7500 women expressed regret at one and two years post-operatively, respectively, and 6.2% sought information about reanastomosis, but only 0.23% obtained a reanastomosis. In this study, the strongest predictor of regret was an age less than 30 at the time of sterilisation.

The psychiatric morbidity before and after sterilisation reveals no difference between those who undergo sterilisation and those who do not. The World Health Organization prospective multicentre study[4] found no significant correlation between the occurrence of psychiatric problems in the follow-up period and tubal sterilisation.

Reports on sexual satisfaction demonstrate that tubal sterilisation has virtually no effect. Shain et al[19] reported no overall differences in sexual satisfaction, coital desire or coital frequency in a five-year period among women who had undergone sterilisation as compared with women whose husbands had had vasectomies or women not planning sterilisation.

REVERSAL

Proper counselling before a surgical contraception procedure should minimise the demand for reversal. Occasionally, however, a woman whose Fallopian tubes have been occluded wishes to recover her fertility. This change of mind may occur if an accident or illness deprives her of one or more of the children she has already borne or if she forms a new relationship with a man who desires children of his own.

Anastomosis of normal tubes that have been occluded under aseptic surgical conditions gives better results than that of tubes blocked as a result of inflammatory disease. The success of reversal is mainly related to the amount of undamaged tube available for anastomosis.

The success rate of tubal ligation reversal is better after mechanical occlusion of the Fallopian tubes than after electrocoagulation, inasmuch as the latter method destroys much more of the tube. Reversal pregnancy rates range from 43% for electrocoagulation, through 59% for the Pomeroy method, and 75% for laparoscopic ring occlusion, to 88% for laparoscopic clip occlusion.

For the time being, the procedure of in vitro fertilisation and embryo transfer offers the best alternative for reversing female surgical contraception.

MALE STERILISATION

GENERAL

The indications for the surgical contraception of men are in many respects similar to those for women, with one important difference. Therapeutic indications in one sense do not exist, because men quite obviously need no protection from the hazards of pregnancy.

The operation, therefore, is undertaken for the protection of the woman's health and to limit the number of children in a given family. The procedure is also safer and simpler than female surgical contraception.[18]

INFORMATION AND LEGISLATION

Voluntary vasectomy, for the purpose of family planning, is readily accessible. Pre-operative information is a decisive factor. The same careful considerations of the consequences of the procedure for women must precede the decision for men. The candidate for the operation should regard the resultant sterility as permanent. Candidates for vasectomy, therefore, should want no further children.

It is most important to inform the patient of the necessity for post-operative ejaculate analyses, because the success of the operation cannot be confirmed without two subsequent demonstrations of azoospermia. Insufficient control of the ejaculate is the most frequent cause of unintended pregnancy after vasectomy.

Voluntary surgical contraception has become a very popular contraceptive method in recent decades. From an estimated world total of only 4 million sterilisations in 1950, in 1991 the number of sterilised men worldwide was estimated to be 50 million. Since then, 60 million men have reportedly undergone vasectomy by means of the no-scalpel method alone. Although precise numbers are currently not available, the present estimate is well over 100 million. The frequency of the use of surgical contraception as a method of contraception varies from country to country. In some countries it is the leading contraceptive method, while in others the non-availability of services or restrictive attitudes, policies and laws prevent large numbers of men and women from effective access to the method. The great majority of surgical contraceptive procedures have been performed in China, India and the United States.

TECHNIQUES

The standard procedure for the occlusion of the vas deferens is surgical, but chemical vas occlusion techniques also exist.

Surgical procedures

Vasectomy

Vasectomy is the standard operation for male surgical contraception. It is a simple one, usually performed under local anaesthesia and without hospitalisation, in 5–15 minutes. Its principle is simply interruption of the continuity of the spermatic duct (vas deferens) in the upper part of the scrotum, as it passes upward from the epididymis.

During the operation, the vas is first identified by palpation. The skin and subcutaneous tissue are then infiltrated with a local anaesthetic, and a short incision is made. Most operators prefer bilateral incisions, one for each vas, but a single midline incision can be used. After the incision is made, the vas is grasped by a clamp, and the soft, fibrous surrounding tissue (the adventitia of the vas) is stripped off for 1 or 2 cm. Resection of a considerable segment of the vas, allowing the two ends to separate widely, increases the reliability of the operation, but makes anastomosis (if reversal is requested) more difficult (Figs 10.7A–E).

Open-ended vasectomy

Another modification of the standard vasectomy procedure is open-ended vasectomy, in which the testicular end of the vas is left unsealed, while the abdominal side is sealed as usual.

In a large comparative trial, men vasectomised with the open-ended technique had about half the rates of epididymal congestion and of painful granuloma as those for men vasectomised with the standard technique.

No-scalpel technique

Researchers in China have developed a vasectomy technique that can be performed with a puncture, not an incision. This technique reduces bleeding, and speeds healing. A specially designed fixing clamp encircles and holds the vas without penetrating the skin. The scrotum and vas sheath are punctured with a sharp-ended haemostat and stretched open. The vas is then lifted out of the scrotum and sealed by ligation or coagulation.[11]

Chemical vas occlusion

This procedure involves no incision. Instead, the scrotum and vas sheath are punctured with a needle, and a chemical occlusion compound of phenol and cyanoacrylate is injected directly into the lumen of each vas. The compound coagulates in the lumen, forming a plug, and the carbolic acid also induces scarring to further close the lumen and block the passage of sperm.

Few subjects have reported complications or discomfort. However, the failure rate of 2.4%, observed in a study of 577 men, is higher than rates with surgical vasectomy techniques.

Reversible vas occlusion

Research is also under way on devices that can be implanted in the vas and later removed to restore fertility. Over 20 different devices have been investigated. Difficulties in inserting the devices and in completely blocking the sperm complicate most of these efforts.

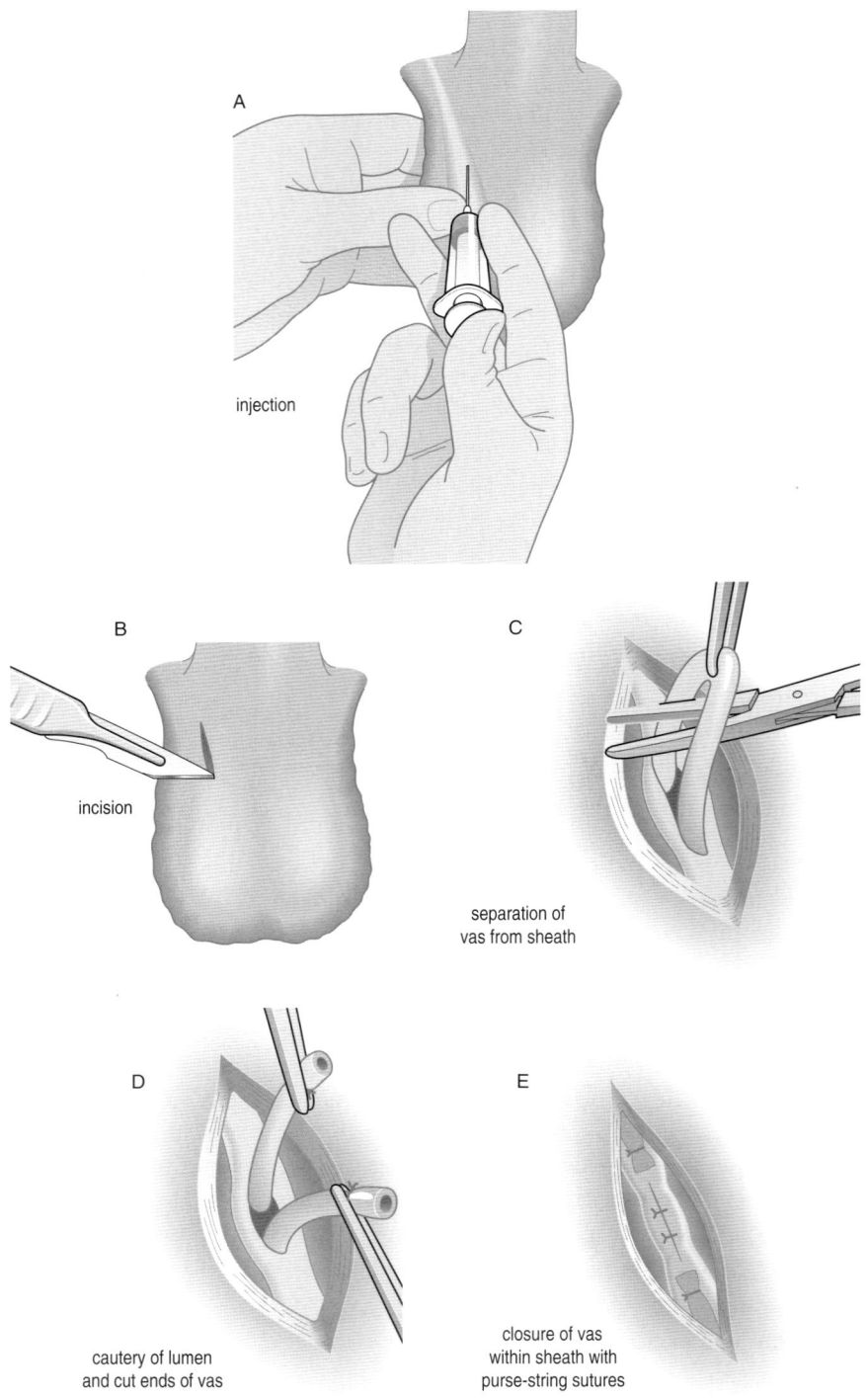

A

injection

B

incision

C

separation of
vas from sheath

D

cautery of lumen
and cut ends of vas

E

closure of vas
within sheath with
purse-string sutures

Fig 10.7 Techniques of vasectomy. **A**, injection; **B**, incision; **C**, separation of vas from sheath; **D**, cautery of lumen and cut ends of vas; **E**, closure of vas within sheath with purse-string sutures. (With permission from the authors[6])

FAILURE

A review of the literature demonstrates that vasectomy is successful in 97.2–99% of all cases, irrespective of the method used. Most statistics indicate a failure rate of less than 1%.[16]

The most frequent cause of undesired pregnancy after vasectomy is unprotected intercourse prior to testing for azoospermia. Spontaneous recanalisation is considered to be a rare event. In individual cases, recanalisation has been observed 5–8 years after vasectomy,[3] but these are extremely rare events.

Post-operative semen analysis

Post-vasectomy semen examination always comprises analysis of the sediment of the ejaculate, in order that single spermatozoa should not be overlooked. Data in the literature range from one to three follow-ups, at intervals of six weeks, for up to one year.

If motile spermatozoa are present in samples taken after six weeks, this is indicative of spontaneous recanalisation, because sperm cells become immotile after three weeks at the latest. The importance of post-vasectomy semen analyses is discussed in broad terms with each patient. The man then signs an agreement that he can be considered infertile only after two consecutive negative semen analyses.

It is therefore surprising how vasectomised patients behave with regard to the requested follow-ups: they are non-compliant rather than compliant. 14–36% of vasectomised men never returned for a semen analysis.[13]

POST-OPERATIVE COMPLICATIONS

Vasectomy is essentially not associated with mortality. Where death has occurred in the developing world it is due to infection, most probably tetanus. The most common complications are for the most part minor, involving wound healing, and occurring in less than 5% of the cases.

The many studies that have been made on the psychological and general health effects of the operation have included questions concerning changes in libido and the sense of general well-being. The statistical data have sometimes been conflicting, but no trend has been discernible that could not be explained on the basis of normal variability over time. Antisperm antibodies may be formed after vasectomy, but these have not been shown to have any deleterious effects in the human. Post-vasectomy pain syndrome is a well-recognised clinical entity. Reports of pain over a long period of time, involving the testis and epididymis after vasectomy, and worsening during sexual activity, lie in the range of 3–8%.[14]

REVERSAL

A small number of men may eventually change their minds and desire restoration of their fertility. The operation of vasovasostomy may then be performed.

The success of this procedure depends in part on the way in which the original operation was conducted.

The success also depends on the skill of the surgeon and on his attention to the finer points of the technique. Using sophisticated surgical techniques and instruments, such as an operating microscope, surgeons have been able to rejoin the vasa and restore fertility in about 50% of selected cases.

Another possible alternative to vasectomy reversal is the freezing and storage of semen prior to vasectomy. The frozen semen can later be thawed and used for artificial insemination.

CONCLUSIONS

From the preceding discussion, it is clear that voluntary surgical contraception has certain advantages that are unique among methods of contraception both in the female and in the male. The simple procedure provides permanent security against conception, without side effects and without any further need for medical supervision. As the only expenditure is for the initial operation, the cost of protection over the years is relatively small.

By comparison, the disadvantages seem relatively small. Trained surgeons and surgical equipment are essential. There are minimal surgical risks, usually in the form of minor operative complications. In some regions, acceptability may be poor due to restrictive attitudes, policies and laws. The generally irreversible character of the procedure presents psychological obstacles for some people, and the operation may subsequently be regretted by a small number of individuals. Practice guidelines on sterilisation by the American College of Obstetricians and Gynecologists and the Royal College of Obstetricians and Gynaecologists were published recently.[2,17]

References

1. Abraham S, Jansen R, Fraser I S et al 1986 The characteristics, perceptions and personalities of women seeking a reversal of their tubal sterilisation. Medical Journal of Australia 145:4–7
2. ACOG practice bulletin 2003 Benefits and risks of sterilization. International Journal of Gynecology and Obstetrics 83: 339–350
3. Alderman P M 1989 General and anomalous sperm disappearance characteristics found in a large vasectomy series. Fertility and Sterility 51:859–862
4. Dube K C, Kumar A, Gupta S P et al 1985 Mental health and female sterilisation: a follow-up. Journal of Biosocial Sciences 17:1–18
5. Fathalla M F 1997 From obstetrics and gynecology to women's health. The road ahead. Parthenon, New York
6. Fathalla M F, Rosenfield A, Indriso C 1990 Surgical contraception. In: Family planning. The FIGO manual of human reproduction, Vol 2. Parthenon, Casterton Hall, pp 143–171
7. Feldblum P J, Hays M, Zipper J, Guzman-Serani R, Sokal D C 2000 Pregnancy rates among Chilean women who had non-surgical sterilisation with quinacrine pellets between 1977 and 1989. Contraception 61:379–384
8. International Medical Advisory Panel (IMAP) 1993 Use of quinacrine pellets for female sterilisation not recommended. IPPF Medical Bulletin 27:4–5
9. Kasliwal A, Farquharson R G 2000 Pregnancy testing prior to sterilisation. British Journal of Obstetrics and Gynaecology 107:1407–1409

10. Lampé L 2000 Operative obstetrics and gynaecology. Medicina Publishers, Budapest

11. Li S Q, Goldstein M, Zhu J, Huber D 1991 The no-scalpel vasectomy. Journal of Urology 145:341–344

12. Ligt-Veneman N G P, Tinga D J, Kragt H, Brandsma G, Van Der Leij G 1999 The efficacy of intratubal silicone in the Ovabloc hysteroscopic method of sterilisation. Acta Obstetricia et Gynecologica Scandinavica 78:824–825

13. Maatman T J, Aldrin L, Carothers G G 1997 Patient noncompliance after vasectomy. Fertility and Sterility 68:552–555

14. Myers S A, Mershon C E, Fuchs E F 1997 Vasectomy reversal for treatment of the post-vasectomy pain syndrome. Journal of Urology 157:518–519

15. Peterson H B, Xia Z, Hughes J M, Wilcox L S, Tylor L R, Trussel J, for the US Collaborative Review of Sterilization Working Group 1996 The risk of pregnancy after tubal sterilization: findings from the US collaborative review of sterilization. American Journal of Obstetrics and Gynecology 174:1161–1170

16. Peterson H B, Xia Z, Wilcox L S, Tylor L R, Trussel J for the US Collaborative Review of Sterilization Working Group 1999 Pregnancy after tubal sterilization with bipolar electrocoagulation. Obstetrics and Gynecology 94:163–167

17. Royal College of Obstetricians and Gynaecologists 2004 Male and female sterilisation. Guideline summary. RCOG Press, London

18. Schwingl P J, Guess H A 2000 Safety and effectiveness of vasectomy. Fertility and Sterility 73:923–936

19. Shain R N, Miller W B, Holden A E G et al 1991 Impact of tubal sterilization and vasectomy on female marital sexuality: results of a controlled longitudinal study. American Journal of Obstetrics and Gynecology 164:763–771

20. Sokal D, Hieu D T, Weiner D H, Vingh D Q, Vach T H, Hanenberg R 2000 Long-term follow-up after quinacrine sterilization in Vietnam. Part I: interim efficacy analysis. Fertility and Sterility 74:1084–1091

21. Sokal D, Hieu D T, Weiner D H, Vingh D Q, Vach T H, Hanenberg R 2000 Long-term follow-up after quinacrine sterilization in Vietnam. Part II: interim efficacy analysis. Fertility and Sterility 74:1092–1101

22. Taylor P J, Freedman B, Wonnacott T et al 1966 Female sterilization: can the woman who will seek reversal be identified prospectively? Journal of Reproduction and Fertility 4:107–215

23. Wilcox L S, Chu S Y, Peterson H B 1990 Characteristics of women who considered or obtained tubal reanastomosis: results from a prospective study of tubal sterilization. Obstetrics and Gynecology 75:661–665

24. Yoon I, Poliakoff S R 1979 Laparoscopic tubal ligation: a follow-up report on the Yoon Falope ring methodology. Journal of Reproductive Medicine 23:76–80

25. Zipper J, Cole L P, Goldsmith A, Wheeler R, Rivera M 1980 Quinacrine hydrochloride pellets: preliminary data on a nonsurgical method of female sterilization. International Journal of Gynaecology and Obstetrics 18:275–279

11

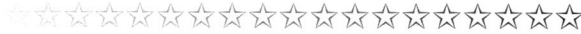

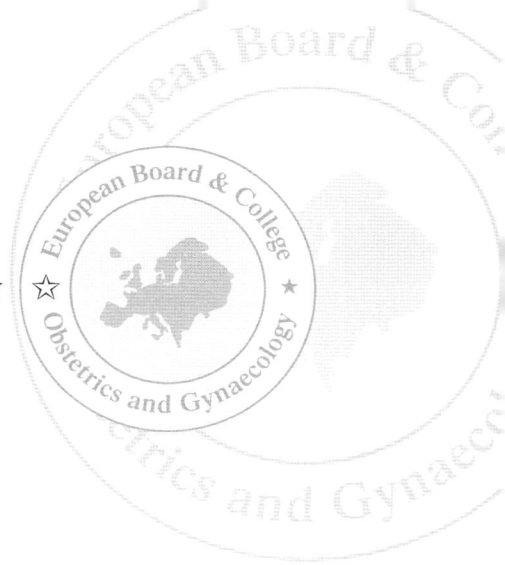

Legal abortion

Marc Bygdeman   Kristina Gemzell Danielsson

ABSTRACT

Most countries in Europe have liberal abortion laws. The most obvious exceptions are Ireland and Poland. However, in some countries legal restrictions and/or the attitude of the population and the medical profession limits the availability of abortion even if abortion is permitted within the law. The most effective and safe surgical methods in the first trimester are vacuum aspiration and in the second trimester are dilatation and evacuation (D&E). In early pregnancy the combination of mifepristone and misoprostol or gemeprost is an attractive medical alternative. In the second trimester either gemeprost or misoprostol, or even better a combination of mifepristone and one of these prostaglandins, are effective and safe alternatives to D&E. The non-invasive nature and simplicity of medical treatment are important aspects. All methods have advantages and disadvantages. The method to be used should be dependent on the choice of the woman, after receiving proper information, and the skill and experience of the providers.

KEYWORDS

Abortion laws, first-trimester abortion, second-trimester abortion, medical abortion methods, vacuum aspiration, dilatation and evacuation, mifepristone, misoprostol, gemeprost

LEGAL SITUATION

CURRENT LAWS

Most countries in Europe have liberal abortion laws. However, because laws are subject to widely varying interpretations by government authorities and by medical personnel and because enforcement is uneven, the literal wording of laws paints an imperfect picture of their impact on medical practice and the actual availability of legal abortion services (Table 11.1).

Moreover, the attitudes of the medical community and the inadequacy of a country's health-care system may limit abortion availability even where services would be legally permissible. Almost all countries in Europe have laws that permit abortion without restriction as to reason. However, all these nations impose an upper gestational limit, which varies from 90 days in Italy to 18 weeks in Sweden. After this time abortion is still permissible but only under limited circumstances. Exceptions are Ireland, where abortion is only allowed to save the life of the woman, and Poland, where the law was revised in 1993 to permit abortion only when a pregnancy threatened the woman's life or health, and on juridical and fetal-impairment grounds. In some countries, such as Portugal, Spain and Switzerland, the law permits abortion to protect the mental health of women. The interpretation of mental health varies. It can encompass the distress suffered by a woman who is raped, the mental distress caused by socioeconomic circumstances or a woman's fear over a medical opinion that the fetus is at risk of being impaired. A few European countries, Great Britain and Finland, permit abortion on socioeconomic grounds. Such laws, which typically permit consideration of a woman's economic resources, her age, her marital status and the number of her living children, are generally interpreted liberally.[16]

LEGAL RESTRICTIONS

The legal status of abortion is not the only or even necessarily the most important factor determining the availability of safe abortion. Some countries require parental authorisation for a minor's abortion. Often abortion services are restricted to government hospitals or other authorised health facilities. Some countries have a mandatory counselling procedure and in some countries such as Germany, Belgium and France the abortion can not be performed until three

Table 11.1 Restrictiveness of abortion law in Europe

Abortion restriction	Countries
To save the woman's life	Ireland
Physical health	Poland
Mental health	Portugal, Spain, Switzerland
Socioeconomic grounds	Finland, Great Britain
Without restriction to reason	Albania, Austria, Belarus, Belgium, Bosnia-Herzegovina, Bulgaria, Croatia, Czech Republic, Denmark, Estonia, France, Germany, Greece, Hungary, Italy, Latvia, Lithuania, Macedonia, Moldova, Netherlands, Norway, Romania, Russian Federation, Slovak Republic, Slovenia, Sweden, Ukraine, Yugoslavia

(Adapted from Rahman A et al 1998 International Family Planning Perspectives 24:56–64)

to six days after the counselling. Countries such as Austria and Lithuania only subsidise abortions performed for medical reasons. The availability of abortion very much depends on the attitude of the medical community and the public. Physicians and community opposition have left parts of Austria and Germany without abortion services even though abortion is legally permitted without restriction to reason. On the other hand, in some countries governmental policy goes beyond permitting abortion to ensure that services are widely available. In Sweden and Denmark, for instance, county health boards are responsible for providing services to all women who decide to have an abortion in the area.[16]

MEDICAL METHODS OF ABORTION

INTRODUCTION

Significant progress in the medical methods used for termination of pregnancies has taken place during the last 30 years. At the beginning of the 1970s intrauterine administration of hypertonic saline and urea was replaced by primary prostaglandins, PGE_2 and $PGF_{2\alpha}$, and later by prostaglandin analogues, such as gemeprost administered vaginally and misoprostol given either orally or vaginally. These compounds stimulate uterine contractility and are especially useful for termination of second-trimester pregnancy and for pre-operative dilatation of the cervical canal. Although abortion can also be induced with these prostaglandins in early pregnancy, the dose required results in a high incidence of undesirable side effects, such as vomiting, diarrhoea and pelvic pain. The development of medical methods for termination of early pregnancy, which were clinically more useful, started in 1982 when Herrman at al[12] showed that the antiprogestin, mifepristone, could terminate pregnancy. Subsequently a number of studies were published in which different daily doses of mifepristone and duration of treatment were used. However, the effect of treatment was disappointing. In general, the frequency of complete abortion was between 60 and 70% in women with an amenorrhoea of less than 56 days. A somewhat higher success rate, around 85%, was found if the treatment was given within the first 10–14 days after the missed menstrual period.[24] An important step forward was made in 1985 with the discovery that mifepristone increased contractility and sensitivity of the myometrium to prostaglandin. The maximum effect was achieved when the prostaglandins were administered 36–48 hours after mifepristone.[3] Pilot studies showed that a sequential regimen of mifepristone and a prostaglandin analogue, such as gemeprost or sulprostone, was highly effective in terminating early pregnancy.[3,4] Subsequently several large multicentre studies were performed with a reported frequency of complete abortion in about 95% of mifepristone pre-treated women.[23] Sulprostone is not used for this purpose any longer since severe cardiovascular complications, including myocardial infarction, were reported. More recently misoprostol has gained increasing use instead. The reason is mainly that misoprostol is available in tablets manufactured for oral use in more than 70 countries for the prevention of gastric ulcers caused by non-steroidal anti-inflammatory drugs. In contrast to gemeprost, misoprostol is also stable at room temperature and is inexpensive. A drawback is that misoprostol is not registered for use during pregnancy, which could cause legal problems in some countries. The use of mifepristone and prostaglandin analogues is not restricted to termination of early pregnancy. Repeated doses of both gemeprost and misoprostol are highly effective in terminating second-trimester pregnancy. If the patients are pre-treated with mifepristone, however, both the duration of labour and the dose of prostaglandin is significantly reduced.

Clinical availability

Mifepristone for termination of pregnancy was first introduced in France in 1989, followed by Great Britain in 1991 and by Sweden and China in 1992. Its use is likely to expand significantly in the near future as it has been recently approved in most European countries as well as in the USA and other countries in different parts of the world. The registered indications for the use of mifepristone in combination with a prostaglandin analogue (gemeprost or misoprostol) are termination of early pregnancy and second-trimester pregnancy, and for mifepristone alone for pre-operative cervical dilatation and labour induction in cases of intrauterine fetal death (Table 11.2).

Table 11.2 Availability and clinical use of antiprogestine (mifepristone) for pregnancy termination in Europe

Country	Year of introduction	Early pregnancy days of amenorrhoea		Pre-operative cervical ripening	Second-trimester pregnancy	Fetal death
		< 49	< 63			
France	1989	*		*	*	*
Great Britain	1991		*	*	*	*
Sweden	1992		*		*	
Germany						
Austria						
Belgium						
Luxembourg						
Netherlands	1999	*		*	*	*
Denmark						
Spain						
Finland						
Greece						
Switzerland						
Russia						
Norway	2000	*		*	*	*
Georgia	2000	*		*	*	*

MODE OF ACTION

Mifepristone

Progesterone is necessary for the establishment and maintenance of pregnancy in all mammals. The corpus luteum secretes large amounts of progesterone, which transforms the endometrium into a secretory state that is receptive to implantation of the embryo. After implantation the placenta takes over the responsibility. Maintenance of pregnancy is dependent on luteal progesterone until the seventh week when the secretion of progesterone by the placenta is sufficient. Progesterone causes relaxation of the myometrium and exerts a suppressive effect on uterine contractions allowing the uterus to accommodate the growing fetus. It is hardly surprising, therefore, that blockage of its receptor leads to abortion.[2] Mifepristone is the only antiprogestin that has reached routine clinical use for termination of pregnancy. It is a derivative of norethisterone with an α-side chain and an 11-β ring substitution, which binds to the progesterone receptor with an affinity five-times as great as that of progesterone and prevents endogenous progesterone from exerting its effect. Mifepristone acts mainly as an antagonist. However, under certain circumstances, e.g. in postmenstrual women whose progesterone concentration is very low, mifepristone will exert a weak agonistic effect on the endometrium following treatment with estrogen. Mifepristone also has a strong antiglucocorticoid effect. After administration of mifepristone, there is a transient rise in the concentration of adrenocorticotropin (ACTH) and subsequent increased levels of cortisol. Clinical experience indicates, however, that this effect is of little significance in the doses of mifepristone used for pregnancy termination. Blockage of the progesterone receptor results in vascular damage, decidual necrosis and bleeding. As mentioned previously, treatment with mifepristone will convey the quiet pregnant uterus into an organ of spontaneous activity with regular uterine contractions. The increased contractility of the uterus can be demonstrated after 24 hours and reaches a maximum 36–48 hours after the administration of mifepristone.[3] The increased uterine activity is due in part to changes in the electrical activity of the myometrium. By reversing the hyperpolarisation of the cell membrane induced by progesterone, the myometrium becomes more sensitive. Mifepristone also reverses the progesterone induced inhibition of gap-junction formation, which is characteristic of the pregnant uterus. With increased formation of gap-junction, the uterus will be able to develop coordinated contractions. The effect of blockade of the progesterone receptor on the blood vessels supplying the decidual and placental beds may result in increased release of PGE_2, which could also contribute to the increased uterine activity. At the same time, as uterine contractility develops, the sensitivity of the myometrium to exogenous prostaglandins will increase five times. It allows the prostaglandin dose used in combination with mifepristone for pregnancy termination to be reduced accordingly and as a consequence prostaglandin-related side effects are also reduced.[3] In addition, mifepristone induces dilatation and softening of the cervix.[2]

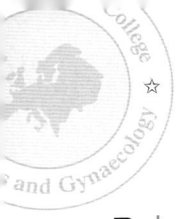

Prostaglandin analogues

The abortifacient effect of prostaglandin analogues is dependent on their effect on uterine contractility. The initial effect is an increase in uterine tonus but with repeated treatment regular uterine contractions will appear. It is probable that a continuing stimulation of uterine contractility is necessary to overcome the blockage of myometrial response caused by progesterone. While an increased endogenous production of $PGF_{2\alpha}$ is the final step in the complicated series of events resulting in uterine activity during spontaneous abortion, it is believed that an increased release of PGE_2 is responsible, together with different cytokines, for the physiological ripening of the cervix at or near term. It is therefore not surprising that treatment with PGE analogues gemeprost and misoprostol have a similar effect. Although an effect on the cervix may have limited importance in early abortion, dilatation of the cervix is essential to permit expulsion of the fetus and placenta in second-trimester abortion and in patients with intrauterine fetal death.

FIRST-TRIMESTER ABORTION

Mifepristone and prostaglandin in combination

Dose of mifepristone

The ideal dose of mifepristone and prostaglandin remains to be established. The recommended dose of mifepristone is 600 mg. Studies in both pregnant and non-pregnant women have shown that the pharmacokinetics of mifepristone are non-linear and that oral administration in single doses higher than 100 mg results in serum concentrations that differ only minimally or not at all. From these data it seemed likely that smaller doses than 600 mg could be effective. In a WHO multicentre study it was also shown that repeated small doses of mifepristone (five doses of 25 mg given at 12-hour intervals) was equally effective as 600 mg mifepristone. In another WHO study it was shown that a single dose of 200 mg was equally effective but if the dose was reduced to 50 mg in combination with gemeprost the complete abortion rate was significantly lower and the rate of continuing pregnancy higher than in women who received 200 mg. It thus seems that 200 mg mifepristone is sufficient and 600 mg mifepristone represents an overdose.[25] It has, however, been suggested in some studies that the pregnancy continuation rate might be lower with the higher dose.

Dose of gemeprost and misoprostol

Gemeprost is available in vaginal suppositories containing 1 mg of the drug, which is also the dose generally used although 0.5 mg seems sufficient. The most commonly used dose of misoprostol is 0.4–0.6 mg given orally. Although misoprostol is only available in tablet form it has also been administered vaginally. Following oral administration, the plasma concentration of misoprostol will rise quickly, peaking approximately 30 minutes after administration and then rapidly declining. In contrast, following vaginal administration the plasma concentration will gradually rise and reach maximum levels after approximately one and a half hours and is thereafter elevated for several hours.[20] From a clinical point of view it is more important that the effect of misoprostol on uterine contractility is also different. The interval from start of treatment to a noticeable effect is significantly shorter following oral administration but more importantly the duration of stimulation is significantly longer following vaginal administration. After oral treatment only a short increase in uterine tonus is recorded while following vaginal administration the initial increase in tone is followed by regular uterine contractions.[9]

Very similar results with regard to plasma levels and effect on uterine contractility have been reported following vaginal administration of gemeprost. Both the pharmacokinetic results and the effect of misoprostol on uterine contractility indicate that vaginal administration could have advantages both with regard to abortifacient efficacy and treatment intervals.

Treatment schedules and clinical outcome

The most used treatment schedules have been 600 mg mifepristone and 36–48 hours later either 1 mg gemeprost administered vaginally or 0.4–0.6 mg misoprostol orally. In three large multicentre studies from France, Great Britain and the World Health Organization, the efficacy and safety of 600 mg mifepristone and 1 mg gemeprost have been evaluated. The treatment was highly effective with a frequency of complete abortion between 94 and 96.3%. The frequency of continuing live pregnancy was between 0.4 and 0.9%. Following treatment approximately 50% of the patients started to bleed at the time of prostaglandin treatment and almost all within four hours thereafter. The mean duration of bleeding varied between 8 and 12 days, but occasionally the bleeding could continue for several weeks.[23] In general, patients reported the bleeding to be more pronounced than that of a normal menstruation. In one study the overall mean blood loss was objectively measured to be 81 ml. However, excessive bleeding requiring therapy is a rare event. A haemostatic surgical procedure was performed in 0.4–1% of the patients and the frequency of blood transfusion varied between 0.1 and 0.9%. In the WHO study there was a significant decrease in haemoglobin value from 125 g L^{-1} pre-treatment to 122 g L^{-1} one week post-treatment but values had returned to their initial levels six weeks post-treatment. Pelvic infection treated with antibiotics was reported in 0.7 to 1.4% of the patients. If the duration of treatment is limited to 49 days gestation, 0.4 mg misoprostol orally in combination with 600 mg mifepristone is equally effective. In several studies a rate of complete abortion of 96–97.5% has been reported (Table 11.3). The failures included persistent pregnancy (1.5%), incomplete expulsion (2.8%) and the need for haemostatic procedure (0.9%). However, if women with pregnancies of up to 63 days are included, oral misoprostol seems less effective than gemeprost. Two large multicentre studies have demonstrated a statistically significant decline in efficacy with increasing length of gestation when misoprostol is administered orally. In both studies, the complete abortion rate was 83–87% in women at 50–56 days and only 78–80% at gestation of 57–63 days.[26] More importantly, the continuing live pregnancy rate increased with the length of gestation in both studies from 1% at 49 days to 9% at 57–63 days. In another study it was demonstrated that 200 mg mifepristone was equally effec-

Table 11.3 Termination of early pregnancy by mifepristone and prostaglandins administered vaginally

	Treatment		
	600 mg mifepristone + 1 mg gemeprost (%)	200 mg mifepristone + 0.8 mg misoprostol (%)	
Outcome	<49days	<49days	50–63 days
Complete abortion	96.5	98.5	96.7
Incomplete abortion	2.3	1.1	2.4
Ongoing pregnancy	0.9	1.4	0.8
Haemostatic surgical procedure	0.8	0.35	
Blood transfusion	0.1	0.15	
Pelvic infection	0.7	3.1	

(Adapted from Ulmann A et al 1992 Acta Obstetricia et Gynecologica Scandinavica 71:278–286; Ashok P W et al 1998 Human Reproduction 13:2962–2965)

tive (97.5% complete abortion) as 600 mg mifepristone in combination with 0.6 mg misoprostol orally up to 49 days' gestation. However, in women with an amenorrhoea between 50 and 63 days, the frequency of complete abortion decreased significantly to 89.1%. In a randomised trial in which 0.6 mg miso-prostol was compared with 0.5 mg gemeprost following 200 mg mifepristone in women with a gestation of up to 63 days, the frequency of complete abortion was the same. However, there were significantly more ongoing pregnancies in the misoprostol group, especially women with an amenorrhoea over 50 days. The study also showed that fewer women required analgesia following misoprostol than following gemeprost (48% vs. 60%) but the need for opiates was similar in both groups. The incidence of nausea and vomiting after misoprostol (47.8% and 21.9%, respectively) was higher than after gemeprost (33.9% and 12%, respectively). Misoprostol has also been administered by the vaginal route. As mentioned previously, pharmacokinetic data and the effect of vaginal misoprostol on uterine contractility indicate that this route may be more effective than the oral one. This has also been confirmed in clinical studies. The combination of 200 mg mifepristone followed by 0.8 mg misoprostol vaginally resulted in 97.5% complete abortion although even women up to nine weeks of amenorrhoea were included.[1] The advantage of the vaginal route was further supported in a randomised study in which 600 mg mifepristone was combined with either 0.6 mg misoprostol orally or 0.8 mg administered vaginally. Mifepristone in combination with vaginal misoprostol was more effective (95% compared with 87%) and in addition the rate of continued pregnancy was 7% with the oral regimen and 1% with the vaginal one.[8] If 0.8 mg of misoprostol is used vaginally the interval between mifepristone and misoprostol administration may be reduced to 24 hours.[18] More recently sublingual administration of misoprostol has been shown to be an effective alternative, which for some women may be a more attractive alternative than the vaginal route (Box 11.1).

Box 11.1   Medical termination of early pregnancy

Licensed regimen
- Mifepristone 600 mg followed by 0.4 mg misoprostol orally 36–48 hours thereafter in pregnancies up to 49 days of amenorrhoea

- Mifepristone 600 mg followed by 1 mg gemeprost vaginally 36–48 hours thereafter in pregnancies up to 63 days of amenorrhoea

Other effective treatments
- Mifepristone 200 mg followed by 0.4–0.6 mg misoprostol orally 36–48 hours thereafter in pregnancies up to 49 days of amenorrhoea

- Mifepristone 200 mg followed by 0.8 mg misoprostol vaginally[24] 36 or 48 hours thereafter in pregnancies up to 63 days of amenorrhoea

---

Clinical management

In countries where mifepristone has been approved, three clinical visits are required. The first visit is for examination, determination of duration of pregnancy, information and start of treatment with mifepristone. Ultrasound scanning is not considered to be an essential prerequisite in all cases. However, it can be a necessary part of pre-abortion assessment particularly where duration of gestation is in doubt or where ectopic pregnancy is suspected. The second visit takes place 36–48 hours later when prostaglandin is given. This visit includes a 4–6 hour period of clinical supervision in connection with the prostaglandin treatment. To reduce patient discomfort it is advisable to give prophylactic analgesia. Drugs like paracetamol and dihydrocodeine are often used. The third visit is normally performed 2–3 weeks after start of treatment to evaluate outcome. In most cases the clinical events, amount and duration of bleeding, and the findings at the gynaecological examination are sufficient to ensure that the woman has had a complete abortion. If there are doubts an ultrasound examination could be helpful, especially if the possibility of an ectopic pregnancy cannot be excluded otherwise. Others have used measurement of hCG before and after treatment and found that a significant decrease was a more reliable method of determining outcome than ultrasound, at least if it was performed only after treatment. Some clinicians in the USA have investigated administrating misoprostol at home and have found it feasible in settings with good communication and transportation so that women can be transferred to hospital if problems occur.[17] Similar studies are also under way in other countries. Both mifepristone and prostaglandins have contraindications that have to be respected. These include women who suffer from adrenal insufficiency or severe asthma or are receiving long-term glycocorticoid therapy. The medical method is also not recommended for use in women who have a history of cardiovascular disease or haemorrhagic disorders, or who receive treatment with anticoagulants. Continuing pregnancies must be terminated surgically since the risk for fetal malformation can not be excluded. Eight cases of malformation have been reported among 71 continuing pregnancies. Five were discovered during pregnancy and the pregnancy was terminated and three were found after delivery. None of the 22 women out of the 71 who were treated with mifepristone and oral misoprostol had any fetal malformation.

Misoprostol alone

In many countries only misoprostol is available and therefore the possibility of using this compound by itself has been tested. In spite of repeated vaginal doses of 0.4 or 0.6 mg the success rate in most studies has been less than sufficient from a clinical point of view. Also, the induction to abortion interval tends to be quite long, in some cases up to several days, and in comparison with the combination of mifepristone and misoprostol seems to be more painful and to give rise to greater gastrointestinal side effects. Uncontrolled use of misoprostol has also been associated with birth defects in pregnancies that continued to term including malformation of the limbs and facial paralysis (Möbius syndrome).

Methotrexate and misoprostol

Another drug that has been tested is methotrexate. Methotrexate is a cytotoxic drug, which has successfully been used for treatment of trophoblastic disease, such as hydatidiform mole and choriocarcinoma and unruptured ectopic pregnancy. Normal trophoblastic tissue is also destroyed by methotrexate and the drug has been used also for induction of abortion in early pregnancy. Methotrexate is usually given in a dose of 50 mg per square metre of body surface area administered by intramuscular injection. Three to seven days later misoprostol (0.8 mg) is administered by the vaginal route. The overall success ranges from 84 to 97%.[6] However, the abortion is often delayed. In 12–35% of women it occurs approximately 20–30 days after the administration of misoprostol. The main concern with methotrexate is its cytotoxic effect on the trophoblast. Limb defects, including shortened limbs and missing digits have been reported in aborted fetuses. Treatment with methotrexate does not seem to be an alternative if mifepristone is available.

SECOND-TRIMESTER ABORTION

As mentioned previously intra- or extra-amniotic administration of primary prostaglandins (PGE_2 and $PGF_{2\alpha}$) for termination of second-trimester pregnancy replaced hypertonic saline and urea at the beginning of the 1970s. The main advantages of prostaglandins were a much shorter induction–abortion interval and a decreased risk for severe complications. The development of prostaglandin analogues, which could be administered vaginally or intramuscularly, represented a further step forward. The non-invasive mode of administration has certainly facilitated the treatment and reduced the risk for complications associated with intrauterine administration. Today gemeprost administered vaginally and more recently misoprostol administrated either orally or vaginally are the drugs mainly used.

Treatment with gemeprost

The treatment schedule for gemeprost is 1 mg repeated every six hours for the first 24 hours. If abortion has not occurred at that time 1 mg gemeprost is administrated three-hourly for the next 12 hours. The mean duration of labour is around 15 hours. Approximately 75% of the women will abort within 24 hours and 95% within 48 hours following start of treatment. The most common side effects are vomiting and diarrhoea, which occur in approximately 25–40% and 25% of women treated, respectively.[21]

Treatment with misoprostol

For misoprostol no definite treatment schedule exists. In most studies vaginal administration has been used and doses between 0.2 and 0.8 mg were given at three, six or 12 hour intervals. For oral administration the dose used is 0.4 mg administered every third hour. The efficacy of misoprostol seems to be equal to that of gemeprost with a mean induction to abortion interval of around 15 hours and a 48-hour successful abortion rate of 95%.[27] In a prospective, randomised, double-blind study, 1 mg gemeprost three-hourly for five doses were compared with 0.2 mg misoprostol vaginally six-hourly for four doses. The treatment was repeated if the patients were not delivered within 24 hours. Delivery within 24 hours occurred in 75.1% of women receiving gemeprost and 74.9% receiving misoprostol. The median time from prostaglandin commencement to delivery was also similar or 13.7 and 16.9 hours, respectively. There was no difference in the incidence of maternal fever >37.8°C, nausea or diarrhoea. The incidence of vomiting in women randomised to misoprostol was significantly lower (13.2% and 34%, respectively).[7]

Mifepristone in combination with prostaglandin

The most effective medical method for termination of second-trimester pregnancy is the combination of mifepristone and gemeprost or misoprostol.[21] As during early pregnancy, the recommended dose is 600 mg administered 36–48 hours prior to prostaglandin treatment but 200 mg seems equally effective. In a randomised study it was demonstrated that the mean interval between start of treatment with gemeprost and abortion decreased from 15.8 hours to 6.8 hours if the patients were pre-treated with 600 mg mifepristone in comparison with placebo (Table 11.4). The dose schedule for gemeprost was the preferred one, 1 mg every six hours and if abortion had not occurred after 24 hours, three-hourly

Table 11.4 Termination of second-trimester pregnancy

Treatment	Abortion within		Mean duration of labour (hours)
	<24 hours (%)	<48 hours (%)	
Mifepristone 200 or 600 mg + 1.0 mg gemeprost repeated adm	96	99	6.6–9.0
Misoprostol 0.4 mg vaginally repeated adm	73	91	15.2
Gemeprost 1.0 mg vaginally	80	95	16.9

(Adapted from Thong K J et al 1992 Prostaglandins 44:65–74; Thong K J, Baird D T 1993 British Journal of Obstetrics and Gynaecology 100:758–761; Gemzell Danielsson K, Östlund E 2000 Acta Obstetricia et Gynecologica Scandinavica 79:702–709; Wong K S et al 2000 Human Reproduction 15:709–712)

over the next 12 hours. In two studies including almost 300 second-trimester pregnancies, this treatment has been further evaluated.

The overall frequency of abortion within 24 hours was 96%. The corresponding figure within 48 hours was 99%. The median time of labour was for primigravidae between 8.2 and 9 hours and for multigravidae between 6.6 and 7.2 hours.[10,22] The duration of pregnancy at the time of treatment had only a marginal influence on the outcome of treatment. Since mifepristone was administered on an out-patient basis and the duration of labour was short, it was now possible to carry out medically induced mid-trimester abortion on a day-care basis in many women. The most common side effects were vomiting (31%) and diarrhoea (5%). In both studies the majority (84–93%) of women received narcotic analgesia for effective pain relief. Only one woman needed blood transfusion and in one patient with a previous history of cone biopsy a posterior cervical tear was found following expulsion. Available data indicate that for gemeprost the incidence of cervical tears is low or around 0.1%. More recently misoprostol has replaced gemeprost for second-trimester abortion. These studies have shown that, e.g. 600 mg mifepristone followed by 0.4 mg misoprostol orally every third hour or 200 mg mifepristone followed by 0.8 mg misoprostol vaginally and thereafter 0.4 mg misoprostol orally every third hour is equally effective and safe as the combination of mifepristone and gemeprost (Box 11.2).[7]

SURGICAL PROCEDURES

The surgical methods mainly used are vacuum aspiration, which has replaced dilatation and curettage (D&C) due to a significant higher complication rate with the latter method, and dilatation and evacuation (D&E). Vacuum aspiration is the method of choice in the first trimester while D&E is the surgical method to be used in second-trimester abortion. Principles of pre-procedural evaluation for surgical abortion are essentially the same as for medical abortion. Routine preoperative assessment includes confirmation of pregnancy, estimation of gestational age and identification through the medical history or physical examination of conditions that might make the procedure more challenging. If the uterus size correlates with the time of last menstrual period, routine pre-operative ultrasonography is not required. Special consideration should be given to conditions

---

Box 11.2 Medical abortion in the second trimester

Licensed treatment
- Mifepristone 600 mg followed 36–48 hours later by 1 mg gemeprost vaginally every third hour up to five doses

Other effective treatments
- Mifepristone 200/600 mg followed 24–48 hours later by 1 mg gemeprost vaginally every sixth hour up to 24 hours, thereafter every third hour

- Mifepristone 200 mg followed 24–48 hours later by 0.8 mg misoprostol vaginally and thereafter 0.4 mg misoprostol orally every third hour up to four times

that may make the procedure more risky, such as obesity, acquired or congenital uterine anomalies, sharp flexion of the uterus, the presence of leiomyomas or previous surgery on the cervix. It is advisable to have a strategy for minimising the risk of post-abortion infective morbidity, which may include either antibiotic prophylaxis or screening for lower genital tract infection with treatment of positive cases. ABO and Rhesus blood groups should be determined and Rh-immunoglobulin given if the woman is Rh-negative at least in pregnancies beyond seven weeks when fetal blood production is established.

FIRST TRIMESTER

Clinical research from all over the world has shown that vacuum aspiration is the safest surgical technique for evacuation of the uterus in the first trimester. With vacuum aspiration the cavity is evacuated by plastic or metal cannulae with diameters ranging from 4 to 10 mm attached to a vacuum source. Electric vacuum aspiration (EVA) employs an electric vacuum pump. With manual vacuum aspiration (MVA), the vacuum is created using a hand-held, hand-activated, 60 ml plastic syringe. The use of MVA is generally restricted to pregnancies less than ten weeks due to an increased frequency of patients with a blood loss greater than 250 ml thereafter. Studies comparing the use of electric pump and manual vacuum technologies have shown equivalent levels of effectiveness and safety in early pregnancy. Vacuum aspiration is preferably performed under local (cervical) anaesthesia since a survey over abortion mortality during more recent years has shown that complications due to general anaesthesia are the most frequent cause of abortion-related deaths in the USA. Administration of non-steroidal anti-inflammatory drugs before surgery augments pain relief. In very early pregnancy, the suction cannula may be inserted without prior dilatation of the cervical canal. Usually, however, an incremental dilatation of the cervix to a diameter in millimetres that approximates to the gestational age of the pregnancy in weeks is needed. The uterine content is then aspirated with a corresponding size cannula. Detection of a 'gritty' sensation as the cannula moves across the endometrial surface suggests completion of the abortion. To check that the abortion is complete, an examination of the fresh tissue aspirate is advisable. In women under the age of 18 years and at gestations of > 10 weeks, or in other circumstances where difficulties in dilating the cervical canal can be expected, it is recommended to pre-treat the patient for cervical ripening. Misoprostol orally 0.4 mg or gemeprost 1 mg vaginally prior to surgery are the most used alternatives. A large number of studies involving over 500 000 women have documented the effectiveness of vacuum aspiration in completely evacuating the content of the uterus—most report an effectiveness rate exceeding 98%.

SECOND TRIMESTER

The preferred surgical technique for abortion from 13 weeks of pregnancy is D&E, although some providers, depending on their experience and the particular case, are able to use vacuum aspiration alone up to 15 weeks. D&E is generally performed under deep sedation or general anaesthesia. D&E requires dilating the cervix and evacuating the uterus using electric vacuum aspiration with a 14–16 mm diameter cannula and forceps. A prerequisite is pre-operative ripening of the cervix and dilatation of the cervical canal. Depending on the length of pregnancy adequate dilatation can require from three hours to a full day. Agents used to prepare the cervix include misoprostol, gemeprost and osmotic dilators, such as laminaria tent. If mifepristone is used it has to be administered 24–36 hours prior to surgery. D&E has to be performed by skilled and experienced physicians who have had a sufficiently large case-load to be safe and effective.

COMPLICATIONS

Mortality

The frequency of complications is related to duration of pregnancy. Large studies from the late 1980s in the USA demonstrate that abortion performed at ten weeks or earlier carries a mortality risk of 0.3 per 100 000 abortions, one of the lowest risks associated with any surgical procedure. This risk rises with each subsequent week of pregnancy: to 0.6 per 100 000 for weeks 11 and 12; 1.8 for weeks 13 to 15; 3.7 for weeks 16 to 20; and 12.7 for week 21 and beyond. Back at the beginning of the 1970s infection and haemorrhage were the leading causes of death. However, during the 1970s anaesthesia complications emerged as one of the leading causes and since 1983 they have become the most frequent cause. Both for the USA and most European countries the overall mortality rate in association with legal abortion is less than 1 per 100 000 procedures.[14]

Morbidity

Immediate complications include haemorrhage, uterine perforation, cervical laceration and anaesthetic problems (Table 11.5). The complications in the early weeks following abortion are infection and long-term effects, mainly reproductive sequelae.[5] Haemorrhage requiring blood transfusion complicates around 1.5 per 1000 abortions overall. The rate is lower for early abortion or 1.2 per 1000 at < 13 weeks and 8.5 per 1000 at > 20 weeks. Uterine perforation is an infrequent but potentially serious complication. The incidence is of the order of 1 to

Table 11.5 Complications following first-trimester vacuum aspiration

Twelve studies in multiple countries; number of patients 210 164	
Type of complication	**Frequency (%)**
Excess bleeding	0.05–4.9
Pelvic infection	0.1–2.2
Cervical injury	0.01–1.6
Uterine perforation	0.02–0.7

(Source: Cates W, Grimes D A 1981 In: Abortion and sterilization. Medical and Social Aspects. Academic Press, London)

4 per 1000 surgical abortions. However, reported rates appear to be underestimated. A report of laparoscopic tubal sterilisation after abortion found the number of unsuspected perforations to be six times the number during the abortion. This increased the rate from 3 to 20 perforations per 1000 operations.[13] Perforation of the uterus especially during second-trimester D&E is a serious complication. In a series from one hospital all patients required laparotomy. Two-thirds had suffered bowel injury and two patients required hysterectomies. The frequency of cervical laceration is difficult to evaluate due to the lack of agreed definitions and substandard data collection. In first-trimester vacuum aspiration it is around 0.5–1.5 per 1000 operations. The corresponding figure with D&E in the second trimester is approximately ten-times higher.[19] Pre-operative ripening of the cervix and dilation of the cervical canal is the best way to reduce this complication. As mentioned earlier, in the USA anaesthetic complications have emerged as the leading cause of abortion-related mortality. Also, the overall complication risk was 1.8-times higher (95%; CI 1.4–2.5) following general anaesthesia in first-trimester termination in one study. Local anaesthesia is safer for second-trimester D&E as well. In a large US cohort study the relative risk of serious complications associated with general anaesthesia was 2.6-times higher (CI 1.4–4.9) than that associated with the use of local anaesthesia. Infection is one of the most common complications, particularly when the abortion is incomplete or the woman harbours pathogens in her cervix. The frequency reported varies considerably. In a large series of suction curettage procedures from Planned Parenthood in New York mild infection occurred in five per 1000 cases and sepsis requiring hospitalisation in two. In another prospective study including 1000 patients undergoing vacuum aspiration 56 patients (5.4%) returned to the hospital due to complications. Of these 48 (4.7%) had signs of infection in spite of the fact that the patients were tested with regard to infection with *Chlamydia trachomatis* and patients with positive cultures were treated. In some settings women often make a single visit to the abortion services and pre-operative screening for sexually transmitted disease is not practical. Hence a number of studies have addressed the potential benefit of prophylactic antibiotics at the time of abortion without pre-operative screening. Several large randomised controlled trials have also shown a significant reduction in post-operative infection rate. Given the potential seriousness of upper genital tract infection and the safety and low cost of peri-operative antibiotic administration use of prophylaxis should be considered.

Reproductive sequelae

Because so many women who have abortions intend to have children in the future, the issue of potential adverse effects on later reproduction is important. Secondary infertility is not increased after suction curettage abortion. It may be the case after a post-abortion infection but this occurs so infrequently that no overall effect is seen. The same seems to be true for the risk of late ectopic pregnancy. Several large case-control studies have shown no increase in risk even after multiple induced abortion. However, abortions complicated by infection or retained products of conception may add to the risk. There seems to be no increased risk for spontaneous abortion after uncomplicated vacuum aspiration while abortion with sharp curettage might increase the risk. An increased risk may also exist in cases of cervical injury or uterine perforation. The risk of multiple evacuations has been suggested. Nevertheless, existing data suggest that repeated induced abortions do not increase the risk. If later pregnancies are carried to delivery, the risk for adverse outcome does not appear to be increased. Such studies have included prematurity, low birth weight and maternal morbidity. This appears to hold true even after multiple abortion.

COMPARISON BETWEEN MEDICAL AND SURGICAL ABORTION

FIRST TRIMESTER

For a true comparison between medical and surgical procedures for termination of early pregnancy, randomised studies are necessary since there are no overall accepted definitions with regard to successful treatment as well as side effects and complications. Such studies are few in number and difficult to perform since many women have already decided at the visit to the hospital which method they want to be used. Except for a very early study, there is only one randomised study comparing mifepristone in combination with gemeprost with vacuum aspiration.[11] In this study there was no significant difference between the surgical and medical method with regard to frequency of complete abortion (98.0 and 98.3%, respectively, for patients up to 49 days of amenorrhoea). There was a tendency for a lower success rate in patients between 50 and 63 days for the medical method but this difference was not statistically significant. Mifepristone and oral misoprostol has been compared with vacuum aspiration in a large comparative trial using the same protocol in which women were allowed to choose the method they preferred. This study, which was performed in three developing countries, showed a higher failure rate for the medical method. Most large studies on vacuum aspiration report a frequency of complete abortion of 98% or more. For mifepristone in combination with a suitable prostaglandin the corresponding figure is between 95 and 98%. These figures indicate that if there is a difference it is marginal. All clinical studies on medical abortion report a longer period of bleeding and an amount of blood loss larger than that normally found for vacuum aspiration. In the randomised study the mean duration was 12.7–13.1 days as compared with 10.2 days for the surgical procedure. In studies where the actual blood loss has been measured the total blood loss exceeded that following surgical abortion even if both blood loss during surgery and during the bleeding days thereafter was included. However, there was no significant difference in haemoglobin change between the two methods in the randomised study. As mentioned previously, in large multicentre studies on medical abortion the frequency of serious haemorrhage requiring haemostatic curettage was around 0.4 and 1.0% and the frequency of blood transfusion between 0.1 and 0.9% (Table 11.6). These frequencies are very similar to those reported for vacuum aspiration. The frequency

Table 11.6 Outcome of medical (mifepristone and gemeprost) and surgical termination of early pregnancy (up to 63 days of amenorrhoea) in large multicentre studies

Outcome	Medical abortion (%)	Vacuum aspiration (%)
Complete abortion	94–96.5	97.9
Heavy bleeding	0.4–1.0	1.1
Pelvic infection	0.7–1.4	0.9
Cervical injury	0	0
Uterine perforation	0	0.2

(Adapted from Ulmann A et al 1992 Acta Obstetricia et Gynecologica Scandinavica 71:278–283; UK Multicentre Trial 1990 British Journal of Obstetrics and Gynaecology 97:480–486; World Health Organization 1993 British Medical Journal 307:532–537; Freedman M A et al 1986 American Journal of Public Health 76:550–554)

of infection is difficult to compare since the definition of infection varies considerably. In the randomised study the frequency of early presumed pelvic infection requiring antibiotic treatment was the same following medical and surgical abortion. However, significantly more women consulted their physicians within eight weeks of abortion because of presumed pelvic infection following vacuum aspiration. Of course, surgical complications, such as cervical laceration and uterine perforation, are not a problem for medical abortion. Side effects including uterine cramps, nausea, vomiting and diarrhoea are far more common among the medical rather than the surgical abortion patients and occur mainly during the first hours following prostaglandin administration when the patient is in the hospital. Obviously all patients having surgical abortion need some form of analgesia during surgery. However, in the randomised study, 2% required parenteral analgesia and 10% oral analgesia post-abortion as compared with 35% and 24% following prostaglandin during the hospital stay. If misoprostol is used parenteral analgesia is only occasionally needed. The mean time taken off work was significantly longer in women who underwent vacuum aspiration but there was no difference in the time taken to return to normal daily activities. The acceptability of the surgical and medical methods has been evaluated in a few studies. Common reasons for women to prefer medical abortion are fear of anaesthesia or surgery and the view that the procedure is less invasive and more 'natural'. A desire to be unconscious and therefore unaware of the procedure and medical abortion being 'too slow' are common reasons for women to prefer vacuum aspiration. If the women are allowed to choose the method to be used, both methods are equally acceptable. The conclusion is that medical abortion does not replace but is an alternative to vacuum aspiration and preferred by many women.[15] In Sweden approximately 50% of eligible women choose medical abortion.

SECOND-TRIMESTER

Old data from the USA showed that D&E had a lower case-fatality rate then medical abortion up to the 20th week of pregnancy.[5] However, at the time for the investigation, the medical method used was intrauterine instillation of saline or prostaglandin. No randomised comparison between modern medical methods, including mifepristone and prostaglandins administered vaginally or orally, has been performed. With the new methods some of the disadvantages of the instillation procedures are substantially reduced, e.g. duration of labour from 24–48 hours to around 6–10 hours. The short duration of labour now allows also second-trimester medical abortions to be performed in day care for many patients. With D&E there is a risk of cervical laceration (0.3–1.0%) and uterine perforation (0.4%) even when performed by skilled gynaecologists. In contrast, uterine rupture and cervical laceration are rare with the new medical methods for late abortion. Women may still prefer D&E due to lower incidence of gastrointestinal side effects, relative absence of pain and not delivering the fetus and placenta. The most important advantages with the medical methods are the non-invasive nature of the procedure and that the experience needed is not much different to that for a delivery. D&E beyond 14 weeks of gestation requires an experienced physician who has a sufficiently large case load to maintain his skill. In countries with a liberal abortion law most abortions are performed before the 12th week of gestation and mid and late second-trimester abortions are few. Under these circumstances concentration of the abortion care to a few centres would be necessary to maintain experience, which might not be a practical solution.

References

1. Ashok P W, Penny G C, Flett G M M, Templeton A A 1998 An effective regimen for early medical abortion: a report of 2000 consecutive cases. Human Reproduction 13:2962–2965
2. Baird D T 2000 Mode of action of medical methods of abortion. Journal of the American Medical Association 55:121–126
3. Bygdeman M, Swahn M L 1985 Progesterone receptor blockage. Effect on uterine contractility in early pregnancy. Contraception 32:45–51
4. Cameron I T, Michie A F, Baird D T 1986 Therapeutic abortion in early pregnancy with antiprogestogen RU486 alone and in combination with a prostaglandin analogue (gemeprost). Contraception 34:459–468
5. Cates W, Grimes D A 1981 Morbidity and mortality of abortion in the United States. In: Hodgson J (ed) Abortion and sterilization: medical and social aspects. Academic Press, London, pp 155–180
6. Creinin M D, Vittinghoff E, Keder L, Darney P D, Tiller D 1996 Methotrexate and misoprostol for early abortion: a multicentre trial. 1. Safety and efficacy. Contraception 53:321–327
7. El-Refaey H, Henshaw K, Templeton A A 1993 The abortifacient effect of misoprostol in the second trimester. A randomized comparison with gemeprost in patients pretreated with mifepristone (RU486). Human Reproduction 8:1744–1746
8. El-Refaey H, Rajasekar D, Abdalla M, Calder L, Templeton A A 1995 Induction of abortion with mifepristone (RU486) and oral or vaginal misoprostol. New England Journal of Medicine 332:983–987
9. Gemzell Danielsson K, Marions L, Rodriguez A, Spur B W, Wong P Y K, Bygdeman M 1999 Comparison between oral and vaginal administration of misoprostol on uterine contractility. Obstetrics and Gynecology 93:275–280
10. Gemzell Danielsson K, Östlund E 2000 Termination of second-trimester pregnancy with mifepristone and gemeprost. Acta Obstetricia et Gynecologica Scandinavica 79:702–706
11. Henshaw R C, Naji S A, Russel I T, Templeton A A 1994 A comparison of medical abortion (using mifepristone and gemeprost) with surgical vacuum aspiration: efficacy and early medical sequelae. Human Reproduction 9:2167–2172
12. Herrmann W, Wyss R, Riondel A, Philibert D, Teutsch G, Sakiz E et al 1982 Effet d'un

steroide anti-progestine chez la femme interruption du cycle et de la grossesse au début. Comptes Rendus de l'Académie des Sciences (Paris) 294:933–938

13. Kaali S G, Szigetvari I A, Bartfai G S 1989 The frequency and management of uterine perforation during first-trimester abortion. American Journal of Obstetrics and Gynecology 161:406–408

14. Lawson H W, Frye A, Atrash H K, Smith J C, Shulman H B, Ramick M 1994 Abortion mortality United States, 1972 through 1987. American Journal of Obstetrics and Gynecology 171:1365–1372

15. MacIsaac L, Darney P 2000 Early surgical abortion: an alternative to and back-up for medical abortion. American Journal of Obstetrics and Gynecology 183:76–83

16. Rahman A, Katzive L, Henshaw S K 1998 A global review of laws on induced abortion. Family Planning Perspectives 24:56–64

17. Schaff E A, Eisinger S H, Stadius L S, Franks P, Gore B Z, Poppema S 1999 Low dose mifepristone, 200mg, and vaginal misoprostol for abortion. Contraception 59:1–6

18. Schaff E A, Fielding S L, Westhoff C, Ellertson C, Eisinger S M, Stadalius L S, Fuller L 2000 Vaginal misoprostol administered 1, 2 or 3 days after mifepristone for early medical abortion. A randomized trial. Journal of the American Medical Association 284:1948–1953

19. Schulz K F, Grimes D A, Cates W Jr 1983 Measures to prevent cervical injury during suction curettage abortion. Lancet i:1182–1184

20. Tang O S, Schweer H, Seyberth H W, Lee S W, Ho P C 2002 Pharmacokinetics of different routes of administration of misoprostol. Human Reproduction 17:332–336

21. Thong K J, Baird D T 1992 A study of gemeprost alone, dilapan or mifepristone in combination with gemeprost for the termination of second-trimester pregnancy. Contraception 46:11–17

22. Tong K J, Baird D T 1993 Induction of second-trimester abortion with mifepristone and gemeprost. British Journal of Obstetrics and Gynaecology 100:758–761

23. Ulmann A, Silvestre L, Chemama L, Rezvani Y, Renault M, Aquillaume C J et al 1992 Medical termination of early pregnancy with mifepristone (RU486) followed by a prostaglandin analogue. Acta Obstetricia et Gynecologica Scandinavica 71:278–283

24. Van Look P F A, Bygdeman M 1989 Antiprogestational steroids: a new dimension in human fertility regulation. Oxford Reviews of Reproductive Biology 11:1–60

25. WHO Task Force on Post-ovulatory Methods of Fertility Regulation 1993 Termination of pregnancy with reduced doses of mifepristone. British Medical Journal 307:532–537

26. WHO Task Force on Post-ovulatory Methods of Fertility Regulation 2000 Comparison of two doses of mifepristone in combination with misoprostol for early medical abortion. British Journal of Obstetrics and Gynaecology 107:524–530

27. Wong K S, Ngai C S W, Yeo E L K, Tang L C H, Ho P C 2000 A comparison of two regimens of intravaginal misoprostol for termination of second-trimester pregnancy: a randomized comparative trial. Human Reproduction 15:709–712

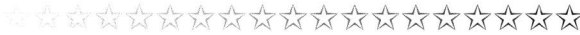

Subject Index

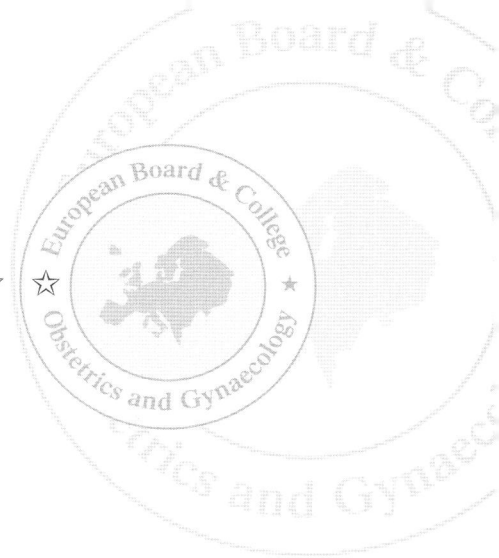

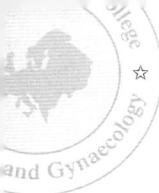